QV 600 LIN   21.99

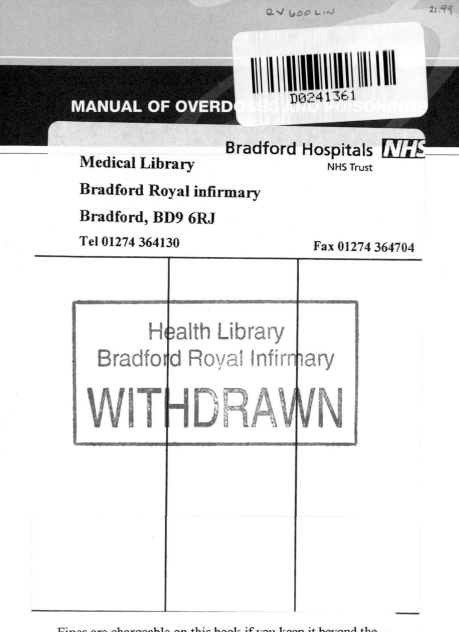

D0241361

MANUAL OF OVERDOSES AND POISONINGS

MANUAL OF OVERDOSES AND POISONINGS

Editors

Christopher H. Linden, M.D.
Associate Professor
Emergency Medicine
Milford Regional
Milford, Massachusetts

James M. Rippe, M.D.
Associate Professor of Medicine
Tufts University School of Medicine
Boston, Massachusetts;
Founder and Director
Rippe Lifestyle Institute
Shrewsbury, Massachusetts

Richard S. Irwin, M.D.
Professor of Medicine
University of Massachusetts Medical School;
Chief, Pulmonary, Allergy, and Critical Care Medicine
UMass Memorial Medical Center
Worcester, Massachusetts

LIPPINCOTT WILLIAMS & WILKINS
A **Wolters Kluwer** Company

Philadelphia • Baltimore • New York • London
Buenos Aires • Hong Kong • Sydney • Tokyo

Acquisitions Editor: Brian Brown
Developmental Editor: Nancy Winter
Managing Editor: Frances Murphy
Marketing Manager: Angela Panetta
Project Manager: Bridgett Dougherty
Design Coordinator: Holly McLaughlin
Production Services: Nesbitt Graphics, Inc.
Printer: R. R. Donnelley & Sons

Library of Congress Cataloging-in-Publication Data

Manual of overdoses and poisonings / edited by Christopher H. Linden, James M. Rippe, and Richard S. Irwin.
    p. ; cm.
  Includes bibliographical references and index.
    ISBN 0-7817-5498-4
  1. Poisoning--Handbooks, manuals, etc. 2. Drugs--Overdosage--Handbooks,
manuals, etc. I. Linden, Christopher H. II. Rippe, James M. III. Irwin, Richard S.
  [DNLM: 1. Poisoning--therapy--Handbooks. 2. Overdose--therapy--Handbooks.
3. Toxicology--Handbooks. QV 607 M294 2005]
RA1215.M36   2005
615.9--dc22
                                                                    20050115081

Care has been taken to confirm the accuracy of the information presented and to describe generally accepted practices. However, the authors, editors, and publisher are not responsible for errors or omissions or for any consequences from application of the information in this book and make no warranty, expressed or implied, with respect to the currency, completeness, or accuracy of the contents of the publication. Application of this information in a particular situation remains the professional responsibility of the practitioner.

The authors, editors, and publisher have exerted every effort to ensure that drug selection and dosage set forth in this text are in accordance with current recommendations and practice at the time of publication. However, in view of ongoing research, changes in government regulations, and the constant flow of information relating to drug therapy and drug reactions, the reader is urged to check the package insert for each drug for any change in indications and dosage and for added warnings and precautions. This is particularly important when the recommended agent is a new or infrequently employed drug.

Some drugs and medical devices presented in this publication have Food and Drug Administration (FDA) clearance for limited use in restricted research settings. It is the responsibility of the health care provider to ascertain the FDA status of each drug or device planned for use in their clinical practice.

10 9 8 7 6 5 4 3 2 1

To purchase additional copies of this book, call our customer service department at (800) 639-3030 or fax orders to (301) 824-7390. International customers should call (301) 714-2324.

Visit Lippincott Williams & Wilkins on the Internet at LWW.com. Lippincott Williams & Wilkins customer service representatives are available from 8:30 am to 6 pm, EST.

CONTENTS

v

Steven B. Bird, M.D.
Assistant Professor of Emergency
Medicine
Department of Emergency Medicine
Division of Medical Toxicology
UMass Memorial Medical Center
55 Lake Avenue North
Worcester, MA 01655

D. Eric Brush, M.D.
Assistant Professor of Emergency
Medicine
Division of Toxicology
UMass Memorial Medical Center
55 Lake Avenue North
Worcester, MA 01655

Ivan E. Liang, M.D.
Staff Physician
Department of Emergency Medicine
Division of Medical Toxicology
UMass Memorial Medical Center
55 Lake Avenue North
Worcester, MA 01655

$\mathcal{T}$he *Manual of Overdoses and Poisonings* is intended for use as a bedside reference and teaching tool for students, residents, fellows, and practitioners who care for patients with toxic or potentially toxic drug and chemical exposures. The first chapter reviews the general approach to the diagnosis and differential diagnosis of poisoning and general principles underlying the evaluation and management of patients with overdose and poisoning. Subsequent chapters focus on specific agents, pharmacological classes of agents, and toxidromes. Chapters are formatted to allow for easy access to information necessary for clinical decision making and include annotated citations of classic and contemporary references as well as details regarding pathophysiology, diagnosis, and treatment. Whenever possible, information is presented in tables and figures.

Although the *Manual of Overdoses and Poisonings* is intended as a stand-alone text, it is related to the fifth edition of *Irwin and Rippe's Intensive Care Medicine* and can be used as an introduction, companion, and study guide for the larger text. Selected chapters from *Irwin and Rippe's Intensive Care Medicine* have been edited, reorganized, condensed, and rewritten in outline format for use in the *Manual of Overdoses and Poisonings*. By focusing on exposures that are common or potentially life threatening, each topic can be covered in depth while keeping the size of the manual small, portable, and readily affordable.

We thank the contributors to this manual for their expertise. We also greatly appreciate the work of our Editorial Director, Elizabeth Porcaro Grady, whose skillful management and oversight has brought the *Manual of Overdoses and Poisonings* to fruition.

Christopher H. Linden, M.D.
James M. Rippe, M.D.
Richard S. Irwin, M.D.

ACKNOWLEDGMENTS

We gratefully acknowledge the love and support of our families, who continue to sustain us and make this work worthwhile.

Christopher H. Linden, M.D.:
Jeanne, Meredith, Martha, and Rebecca

James M. Rippe, M.D.:
Stephanie, Hart, Jaelin, Devon, and Jamie

Richard S. Irwin, M.D.:
Diane, Rachel, Sara, Jamie, Rebecca, Andy K, Andy Mc,
John, Benjamin, Jacob, Isaac, Truman, and Emmett

GENERAL CONSIDERATIONS IN THE EVALUATION AND TREATMENT OF POISONING

Steven B. Bird

I. GENERAL PRINCIPLES. Goals and priorities in the evaluation and treatment of the patient with a chemical exposure and potential poisoning include:

A. Recognition (Diagnosis) of Poisoning

B. Identification of the Offending Agents

C. Prediction of Potential Toxicity

D. Assessment of Severity

E. Provision of Supportive Care

F. Prevention of Chemical Absorption

G. Prevention or Reversal of Poisoning by the Use of Antidotes

H. Enhancement of Chemical Elimination

I. Safe Disposition

J. Prevention of Reexposure

II. EVALUATION

A. Recognition of Poisoning
1. Diagnosis is often made on the basis of a history of chemical exposure, a clinical course consistent with poisoning, and exclusion of other causes.
2. Poisoning should always be considered in patients with metabolic abnormalities (especially acid-base disturbances), gastroenteritis, or changes in mental status of unclear cause.
3. Signs and symptoms of poisoning typically develop within minutes to an hour of an acute exposure, progress to a maximum within several hours, and gradually resolve over a period of hours to a few days.

B. Identification of the Offending Agent
1. Poison Centers, Poisindex, Material Data Safety Sheets (MSDS), and Internet search engines can be used to identify the contents of unknown pills and products.

2. Plants, mushrooms, venomous insects, reptiles, and other animals can be identified by experts from local specialty societies, colleges, botanical gardens, and zoos.

3. The mental status and vital signs provide the most useful information for identifying the cause of poisoning by an unknown agent. Using these parameters, the physiologic state can usually be characterized into one of four categories and a differential diagnosis can then be formulated (Table 1-1).

  a. Common causes of seizures are tricyclic antidepressants, cocaine, amphetamines, antihistamines, theophylline, and isoniazid (INH).

   (1) Seizures are usually generalized but carbon monoxide, hypoglycemic agents, and theophylline can cause focal seizures.

   (2) Central nervous system (CNS) hemorrhage is a complication of poisoning, and a CT scan of the brain should be obtained if focal signs and symptoms are present.

  b. Laboratory studies

   (1) Anion and osmolar gaps and serum ketone and lactate levels can provide important diagnostic clues (Fig. 1-1).

   i. The anion gap, calculated by subtracting the serum chloride and bicarbonate concentrations from the serum sodium concentration, is normally 13 ± 4 mEq/L.

   ii. The serum osmolality is normally 290 ± 10 mOsm/kg of H_2O, and the normal osmolar gap—the difference between the serum osmolality (measured by freezing point depression) and the calculated serum osmolality—is 5 ± 7 mOsm/kg.

   ▪ The serum osmolality is calculated by doubling the serum sodium concentration and adding the result to the serum glucose and blood urea nitrogen (BUN) concentrations (assuming that all concentrations are measured in millimoles per liter).

   ▪ If glucose and BUN are measured in milligrams per deciliter, dividing these values by 18 and 3, respectively, will give their approximate concentrations in millimoles per liter.

   ▪ The approximate concentration of low molecular weight solutes that increase the serum osmolality by 1 mOsm/kg of H_2O, calculated on the basis of their molecular weights, is shown in Table 1-2.

   ▪ Toxic solute concentrations can be estimated by multiplying the concentration listed in Table 1-2 by the excess osmolar gap.

   (2) Pregnancy testing is recommended in women of childbearing age.

   (3) Hypokalemia can be caused by barium salts, β agonists, diuretics, methylxanthines, and toluene.

   (4) Hyperkalemia can be caused by α-agonists, β-blockers, cardiac glycosides, and fluoride.

   (5) Potential hepatotoxins include acetaminophen, ethanol, halogenated hydrocarbons (e.g., carbon tetrachloride), heavy metals, and mushrooms (e.g., *Amanita* species).

   (6) Renal dysfunction can be caused by ethylene glycol, agents causing rhabdomyolysis or hemolysis, nonsteroidal antiinflammatory drugs (NSAIDs), and toluene.

TABLE 1-1 Differential Diagnosis of Poisoning Based on Physiologic Abnormalities, Underlying Mechanisms, and Specific Causes

	Physiologic state		
Excited (CNS stimulation with increased vital signs)	**Depressed (CNS depression with decreased vital signs)**	**Discordant (mixed CNS and vital sign abnormalities)**	**Normal**
Sympathomimetics	**Sympatholytics**	**Asphyxiants**	Nontoxic exposure
Amphetamines	α-Adrenergic antagonists	Carbon monoxide	**Psychogenic illness**
Bronchodilators (β agonists)	Angiotensin-converting	Cyanide	**Toxic time bombs**
Catecholamine analogues	enzyme inhibitors	Hydrogen sulfide	Acetaminophen
Cocaine	β-Adrenergic blockers	Inert (simple) gases	Agents that form concretions
Decongestants	Calcium-channel blockers	Irritant gases	*Amanita phalloides* and
Ergot alkaloids	Clonidine gestants	Methemoglobinemia	related mushrooms
Methylxanthines	Cyclic antidepressants	Oxidative phosphorylation inhibitors	Anticholinergics
Monoamine oxidase inhibitors	Decongestants (imidazolones)	Herbicides (nitrophenols)	Cancer therapeutics
Thyroid hormones	Digitalis	**Membrane active agents**	Carbamazepine
Anticholinergics	Neuroleptics	Amantadine	Chloramphenicol
Antihistamines	**Cholinergics**	Antiarrhythmics	Chlorinated hydrocarbons
Atropine and other	Bethanechol	Beta-blockers	Digitalis preparations
belladonna alkaloids	Carbamate insecticides	Cyclic antidepressants	Dilantin kapseals
Cyclic antidepressants	Echothiophate	Fluoride	Disulfiram
Cyclobenzaprine	Myasthenia gravis therapeutics	Heavy metals	Enteric-coated pills
Muscle relaxants	Nicotine	Lithium	Ethylene glycol
Mydriatics (topical)	Organophosphate insecticides	Local anesthetics	Heavy metals
Nonprescription sleep aids	Physostigmine	Meperidine/propoxyphene	Immunosuppressive agents
Parkinsonian therapeutics	Pilocarpine	Neuroleptics	Lithium
Phenothiazines	Urecholine	Quinine (antimalarials)	Lomotil (atrophine and
Plants/mushrooms	**Opioids**	**AGMA[a] inducers**	diphenoxylate)
Hallucinogens	Analgesics	Alcoholic ketoacidosis	Methanol
LSD and tryptamine	Antidiarrheal drugs	Ethylene glycol	Methemoglobin inducers
derivatives	Fentanyl and derivatives	Methanol (formaldehyde)	(some)

(continued)

TABLE 1-1 Differential Diagnosis of Poisoning Based on Physiologic Abnormalities, Underlying Mechanisms, and Specific Causes (*Continued*)

Excited (CNS stimulation with increased vital signs)	Depressed (CNS depression with decreased vital signs)	Discordant (mixed CNS and vital sign abnormalities)	Normal
Marijuana	Heroin	Paraldehyde	Monoamine oxidase inhibitors
Mescaline and amphetamine	Opium	Metformin (biguanide hypoglycemics)	Paraquat
derivatives	**Sedative-hypnotics**	Salicylate	Opioids
Psilocybin mushrooms	Alcohols	Toluene	Organophosphate
Phencyclidine	Anticonvulsants	Valproic acid	insecticides (some)
Withdrawal syndromes	Barbiturates	**CNS syndromes**	Podophyllin
β-Adrenergic blockers	Benzodiazepines	Disulfiram	Salicylates
Clonidine	Bromide	Extrapyramidal reactions	Sustained-release formulations
Cyclic antidepressants	Ethchlorvynol	Isoniazid (GABA lytic)	Thyroid hormone
Ethanol	Gamma hydroxybutyrate	Neuroleptic malignant syndrome	synthesis inhibitors
Opioids	Glutethimide	Serotonin syndrome	Viral antimicrobials
Sedative-hypnotics	Methyprylon	Solvent (hydrocarbon) inhalation	
	Muscle relaxants	Strychnine (glycinergic)	

Source: Irwin RS, Rippe JM. *Irwin and Rippe's Intensive Care Medicine*, 5th ed. Philadelphia: Lippincott Williams & Wilkins, 2003:1328.
[a]Low-lactate increased anion gap metabolic acidosis.

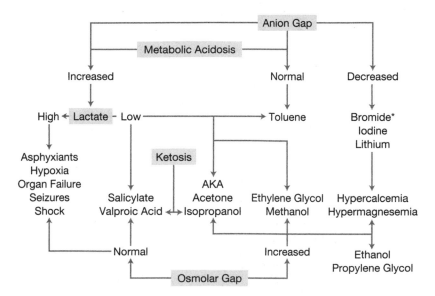

Figure 1-1. Use of the anion gap, osmolar gap, and serum lactate and ketones in the diagnosis of poisoning.

*See text for other (rare) causes; AKA, alcoholic ketoacidosis.

Source: Irwin RS, Rippe JM. *Irwin and Rippe's Intensive Care Medicine,* 5th ed. Philadelphia: Lippincott Williams & Wilkins, 2003:1330.

TABLE 1-2	Effects of Some Solutes on Serum Osmolality
Solute	**Approximate concentration required to increase serum osmolality by 1 mOsm/kg**
Alcohols, glycols, and ketones	
Acetone	5.8 mg/dL
Ethanol	4.6 mg/dL
Ethylene glycol	5.2 mg/dL
Isopropanol	6.0 mg/dL
Methanol	2.6 mg/dL
Propylene glycol	7.6 mg/dL
Electrolytes	
Calcium	4.0 mg/dL (1 mEq/L)
Magnesium	2.4 mg/dL (1 mEq/L)
Sugars	
Mannitol	18 mg/dL
Sorbitol	18 mg/dL

Source: Irwin RS, Rippe JM. *Irwin and Rippe's Intensive Care Medicine,* 5th ed. Philadelphia: Lippincott Williams & Wilkins, 2003:1330.

    c. Electrocardiographic (ECG) findings

        (1) Ventricular tachydysrhythmias can result from myocardial irritation (enhanced automaticity) or reentry mechanisms (resulting from delayed cardiac conduction).

            i. Myocardial irritants include sympathomimetics, cardiac glycosides, and halogenated hydrocarbons.

            ii. Delayed cardiac repolarization and depolarization are manifested by an increased QRS duration and prolonged QTc interval, respectively. Causes include amantadine, types I and III antidysrhythmics (see Chapter 4), β-blockers, fluoride, heavy metals (e.g., arsenic, thallium), magnesium, normeperidine, organophosphate insecticides, potassium, cyclic antidepressants, antipsychotics, quinine, and related antimalarials.

        (2) Atrioventricular block and bradydysrhythmias can be caused by β-blockers, calcium channel blockers, cardiac glycosides, organophosphate insecticides, and phenylpropanolamine.

    d. Radiographic findings

        (1) Radiopaque agents are identified by the mnemonic CHIPE (chlorinated hydrocarbons, calcium salts, heavy metals, iron salts, iodinated compounds, phenothiazines, packets of drugs, and enteric-coated tablets).

        (2) The chest radiograph may demonstrate infiltrates following inhalation of irritant gases (e.g., chlorine, noncardiogenic pulmonary edema), fumes (e.g., metal oxides), vapors (e.g., isocyanates), and some ingestions (e.g., paraquat, salicylates).

    e. Toxicology testing

        (1) Comprehensive toxicology screens are often neither clinically useful nor cost effective. They are not immediately available, can detect only a small fraction of all chemicals, and are not always reliable.

            i. A false-negative result can occur when the toxin is not included in the assay panel or when the concentration of the toxin is below the level of detection by the assay.

            ii. The physician should speak directly with the laboratory technician to determine whether the assay is appropriate for the toxin being considered.

        (2) Quantitative acetaminophen and salicylate concentrations should be obtained in all patients suspected of overdose.

C. Prediction of Potential Toxicity

    1. Depends on dose and time elapsed since exposure as well as on identity of the exposure agent.

    2. Assume a worse-case scenario (maximal possible dose, maximum toxicity from estimated dose)

    3. Criteria for a nontoxic exposure

        a. Patient is asymptomatic by both history and physical examination.

        b. Amount and identity of all chemicals and time of exposure are known with high degree of certainty.

    c. Exposure dose is less than the smallest dose known or predicted to cause toxicity.

    d. Time elapsed since exposure is greater than the longest known or predicted interval between exposure and peak toxicity.

  4. Beware of agents causing delayed toxicity (toxic time bombs; Table 1-1).

D. Assessment of Severity

  1. The severity of poisoning is primarily determined by findings on physical examination (Table 1-3).

  2. The number and type of ancillary tests required to assess metabolic or organ function is determined by clinical severity and by the nature of the exposure.

    a. Patients who are symptomatic or suicidal should have serum electrolytes, BUN, creatinine, and glucose measurements; urinalysis; and 12-lead ECG.

    b. Patients with grade 2 or greater stimulant or depressant poisoning (Table 1-3) should also have a complete blood count; coagulation studies; determination of serum amylase, calcium, magnesium, creatine phosphokinase, hepatic enzyme levels; and a chest radiograph.

    c. Agents for which quantitative measurements are necessary or desirable for optimal patient management include acetaminophen, acetone, alcohols, antiarrhythmics, antiepileptics, barbiturates, carbon monoxide, digoxin, electrolytes (including calcium and magnesium), ethylene glycol, heavy metals, lithium, salicylate, and theophylline.

TABLE 1-3	Physiologic Grading of the Severity of Poisoning	
	Signs and symptoms	
Severity	**Stimulant poisoning**	**Depressant poisoning**
Grade 1	Agitation, anxiety, diaphoresis, hyperreflexia, mydriasis, tremors	Ataxia, confusion, lethargy, weakness, verbal, able to follow commands
Grade 2	Confusion, fever, hyperactivity, hypertension, tachycardia, tachypnea	Mild coma (nonverbal but responsive to pain); brainstem and deep tendon reflexes intact
Grade 3	Delirium, hallucinations, hyperpyrexia, tachyarrhythmias	Moderate coma (respiratory depression, unresponsive to pain); some but not all reflexes absent
Grade 4	Coma, cardiovascular collapse, seizures	Deep coma (apnea, cardiovascular depression); all reflexes absent

Source: Irwin RS, Rippe JM. *Irwin and Rippe's Intensive Care Medicine,* 5th ed. Philadelphia: Lippincott Williams & Wilkins, 2003:1328.

III. TREATMENT

A. Provision of Supportive Care

1. Supportive care includes monitoring (e.g., behavioral, cardiac rhythm, pulse oximetry, urine output, vital signs) and is the primary therapy for most poisoned patients.

2. Respiratory care

   a. Prophylactic intubation may be required for patients with CNS depression to prevent aspiration of gastric contents and is recommended for those who cannot respond to and by voice or who are unable to sit upright and drink fluids without assistance.

   b. Using the gag reflex to assess the need for intubation should be abandoned. Many normal individuals have an absent gag reflex and many comatose patients will gag if sufficiently stimulated and yet be unable to protect their airways. In addition, attempting to elicit a gag reflex may itself induce vomiting and cause aspiration in a patient with an altered mental state.

   c. Prophylactic or therapeutic intubation may also be required for patients with extreme behavioral or physiologic stimulation who require aggressive pharmacologic therapy with sedative, antipsychotic, anticonvulsant, or paralyzing agents.

   d. Even in comatose patients, pretreatment with a sedative and neuromuscular blocking agent can facilitate intubation.

   e. Extracorporeal membrane oxygenation (ECMO) and extracorporeal CO_2 removal (ECCOR), cardiopulmonary bypass, partial liquid fluorocarbon ventilation, hyperbaric oxygen, nitric oxide, and synthetic surfactants should be considered in patients with reversible poisoning who cannot otherwise be adequately oxygenated or ventilated.

3. Cardiovascular therapy

   a. Maintenance or restoration of a normal blood pressure, pulse, and sinus rhythm are the goals of therapy.

   b. Invasive hemodynamic (e.g., arterial, central venous, pulmonary artery pressure) monitoring may be necessary for optimal treatment.

   c. Hypotension (in the absence of an extremely fast or slow heart rate) should initially be treated with intravenous normal saline. A direct-acting vasopressor with inotropic activity, (e.g., norepinephrine, epinephrine, or high-dose dopamine) should be infused for refractory hypotension.

   d. Hypertension often responds to nonspecific sedation with a benzodiazepine. If severe or if chest pain, ECG evidence of ischemia, headache, papilledema, or encephalopathy is present, specific therapy is indicated. A nonselective sympatholytic (e.g., labetalol) or the combination of an α-blocker and a peripheral vasodilator (e.g., esmolol with nitroprusside) is preferred in patients with sympathomimetic poisoning. A vasodilator alone can be used if hypertension is associated with a normal heart rate or reflex bradycardia.

   e. The treatment of ventricular tachydysrhythmias includes correction of electrolyte and metabolic abnormalities. Lidocaine is generally safe.

(1) Sodium bicarbonate, hypertonic saline, or hyperventilation may be effective for wide-complex tachycardias caused by antiarrhythmics, cyclic antidepressants, and possibly other membrane-active agents.

(2) Procainamide and other IA and IC antiarrhythmics (see Chapter 4) are contraindicated in patients with prolonged QRS and QT intervals.

   f. Symptomatic bradycardia should be treated with atropine and dopamine or epinephrine. When it is the result of β-blocker or calcium channel blocker poisoning, treatment includes intravenous calcium, glucagons, and glucose-insulin-potassium infusion.

   g. External or internal electrical cardiac pacing and intraaortic balloon pump counterpulsation or cardiopulmonary bypass should be considered in patients who are unresponsive to routine therapy.

4. Neuromuscular therapy

   a. Treatment of neuromuscular hyperactivity is necessary to prevent or limit rhabdomyolysis and thermogenesis (hyperthermia).

   b. Hyperactivity from sympathomimetic or hallucinogen poisoning and drug withdrawal should initially be treated with sedation using benzodiazepines. Benzodiazepines are preferred to neuroleptics (e.g., chlorpromazine, haloperidol) because the latter are more likely to cause hypotension.

   c. Seizures are treated with benzodiazepines and barbiturates.

   d. Administration of pyridoxine is necessary to stop seizures caused by INH.

   e. Paralyzing (neuromuscular blocking) agents should be given to patients who fail to respond to sedatives and anticonvulsants. During such therapy, seizures should continue to be monitored (by electroencephalograph) and treated to prevent permanent neurologic damage.

B. Prevention of Chemical Absorption

1. Decontamination is recommended in all patients who present within an hour or two of exposure unless the exposure is clearly nontoxic.

2. Body surfaces exposed to acids or alkali should be immediately irrigated until the pH is between 5 and 8.

3. Oral activated charcoal is the recommended method of decontamination for most ingestions. The optimal dose is at least 10 times the weight of the ingested toxin or a maximum of 1 to 2 g/kg of body weight. Activated charcoal is not recommended for ingestions of alkali, acids, or hydrocarbons with low systemic toxicity. It does not effectively bind inorganic salts (e.g., iron, lithium).

4. The routine use of gastric lavage or syrup of ipecac is not supported by current data.

5. Whole bowel irrigation (WBI), the oral administration of large volumes (0.5 L/h in children aged 6 to 12 years and 2 L/h for older patients) of a balanced electrolyte solution (e.g., Golytely) until the rectal effluent is clear may be useful for ingestions of enteric-coated or sustained-release formulations, potentially toxic foreign bodies, and agents that are poorly adsorbed by activated charcoal.

6. Endoscopy can be used to remove foreign bodies or break up drug masses in the stomach. It should be reserved for patients with severe or potentially lethal poisoning, such as those with large amounts of heavy metal visible in the stomach on radiography and those who deteriorate or have rising drug levels despite attempts at gut decontamination by other methods.

  7. Cathartics have not been shown to prevent absorption but they may be useful to prevent constipation from charcoal. Cathartics are contraindicated in patients with caustic ingestions, not recommended in patients with renal insufficiency, and unnecessary in patients with diarrhea.

C. Prevention or Reversal of Poisoning by the Use of Antidotes
  1. Selective antidotes (see Table 1-4) act by competing with chemicals for target sites or metabolic activation pathways, by neutralizing them as a

| **TABLE 1-4** | **Chemicals and Toxic Syndromes with Specific Antidotes** |

Agent/condition	Antidotes
Acetaminophen	N-Acetylcysteine
Anticholinergic poisoning	Physostigmine
Anticoagulants	Phytonadione (vitamine K), protamine
Benzodiazepines	Flumazenil
β-Adrenergic antagonists	Glucagon, calcium salts
Calcium channel blockers	Calcium salts, glucagons
Carbon monoxide	Oxygen, hyperbaric oxygen
Cholinergic syndrome	Atropine, pralidoxime
Cyanide	Nitrites, thiosulfate, hydroxycobal
Digoxin (digitalis)	Fab antibody fragments, magnesium
Dystonic reactions	Benztropine, diphenhydramine
Ethylene glycol	Ethanol, 4-methylpyrazole; pyridoxine, thiamine
Envenomations (arthropod, snake)	Antivenins
Fluoride	Calcium and magnesium salts
Heavy metals (arsenic, mercury, lead)	British antilewisite (dimercaprol), dimercaptosuccinic acid, D-penicillamine, calcium disodium, ethylenediaminetetraacetic acid
Hydrogen sulfide	Oxygen, nitrites
Iron	Deferoxamine
Isoniazid (hydrazines)	γ-Aminobutyric acid agonists, pyridoxine
Methanol	Ethanol, 4-methylpyrazole; folate
Methemoglobinemia	Methylene blue
Opioids	Naloxone, nalmefene, naltrexone
Sympathomimetics	Adrenergic blockers
Vacor (N-3-pyridylmethyl-N′-p-nitrophenylurea)	Nicotinamide (niacinamide)

Source: Irwin RS, Rippe JM. *Irwin and Rippe's Intensive Care Medicine,* 5th ed. Philadelphia: Lippincott Williams & Wilkins, 2003:1332.

result of antibody–antigen reactions or by binding them (i.e., chelation), by promoting their metabolic detoxification, and by antagonizing their autonomic effects through activation or inhibition of opposing neuronal pathways.

2. Nonselective antidotal therapy includes correcting metabolic derangements and enhancing nonmetabolic chemical elimination.

3. The safe use of selective antidotes requires knowledge of their specific indications, contraindications, dosing, and potential complications (see subsequent chapters for details).

D. Enhancement of Chemical Elimination

1. The elimination of some toxins by nonmetabolic routes can be enhanced by diuresis, alkalization of the urine, multiple-dose activated charcoal (MDAC), WBI, and extracorporeal techniques.

2. The choice of technique is dependent on the actual or predicted severity of poisoning and its reversibility, the function of intrinsic detoxification mechanisms, and the potential risks of the intervention and its efficacy in removing the toxin.

3. Urinary alkalinization (urine pH above 7.5) can enhance the renal excretion of acidic chemicals (chlorphenoxyacetic acid herbicide 2,4-D, chlorpropamide, diflunisal, fluoride, phenobarbital, sulfonamides, and salicylates) by ion trapping.

   a. An alkalinizing solution for infusion can be created by adding 134 mEq (three ampules) of sodium bicarbonate to 1 liter of D_5W. It is administered at the same rate as the desired urine output.

   b. Acid-base, electrolyte parameters (particularly potassium and magnesium), and respiratory function must be carefully monitored.

4. MDAC can enhance the elimination of previously absorbed chemicals by binding them within the gastrointestinal (GI) tract as they are excreted in the bile, secreted by the stomach or intestine, or passively diffused back into the gut lumen. MDAC can also enhance the elimination of agents administered parenterally. The recommended dose of activated charcoal is 0.5 to 1 g/kg every 2 to 4 hours. Cathartics can cause water and electrolyte imbalance and are recommended only with the initial dose of charcoal.

5. Extracorporeal methods include hemodialysis, hemoperfusion, hemofiltration, plasmapheresis, peritoneal dialysis, and exchange transfusion. Hemodialysis can effectively remove barbiturates, bromide, chloral hydrate, ethanol, ethylene glycol, isopropyl alcohol, lithium, methanol, procainamide, theophylline, salicylates, and possibly heavy metals. Patients should be monitored for a rebound (increase) in blood levels and clinical toxicity after the termination of extracorporeal therapies.

E. Safe Disposition

1. Admission to the intensive care unit (ICU) is recommended for patients with coma grade 2 or greater, hypotension (systolic pressure of 80 mm Hg or lower), respiratory depression (P_{CO_2} >45 mm Hg or intubated), a nonsinus cardiac rhythm (including second- or third-degree atrioventricular block), seizures, extremes of temperature, severe hypertension,

agitation, hallucinations, or metabolic abnormalities and those who require antidotal or enhanced elimination therapy.
   2. Patients who are less ill, stable, or asymptomatic and who need close or continuous visual observation (e.g., one-to-one suicide precautions) and close or continuous monitoring of cardiac rhythm and vital signs can be admitted to an intermediate care unit, telemetry unit, or emergency department observation unit.
   3. Suicidal patients require psychiatric evaluation, disposition, and follow-up.

F. Prevention of Reexposure
   1. The environment of children should be poison proofed.
   2. Substance abusers (recreational users and addicts) should be counseled regarding attendant medical risks and given the opportunity for rehabilitation through referral for behavior modification, supervised withdrawal, and abstinence or maintenance therapy.
   3. Adults with accidental poisoning should be educated regarding the safe use of drugs and other chemicals.
   4. Workplace exposures should be reported to the appropriate governmental agency (i.e., Occupational Safety and Health Administration and/or local health department), and workers should be warned to avoid reexposure.

Selected Readings
Bond GR. Home syrup of ipecac use does not reduce emergency department use or improve outcome. *Pediatrics* 2003;112:1061–1064.
   This study suggests that no reduction in resource utilization or improvement in patient outcome results from the use of syrup of ipecac at home.

Goldfrank LR, Flomenbaum NE, Lewin NA, et al. Vital signs and toxic syndromes. In: Goldfrank KR, Flomenbaum NE, Lewin NA, et al., eds. *Toxicologic emergencies,* 7th ed. New York, New York: McGraw-Hill, 2002.
   A discussion of the classic clinical manifestations of a variety of toxicologic exposures.

Krenzelok E, Vale A. Position statements: gut decontamination. American Academy of Clinical Toxicology, European Association of Poisons Centres and Clinical Toxicologists. *J Toxicol Clin Toxicol* 1997;35:695–786.
   This review discusses the role of various gut decontamination therapies in poisoned patients.

Nice A, Leikin JB, Maturen A, et al. Toxidrome recognition to improve efficiency of emergency urine drug screens. *Ann Emerg Med* 1988;17:676–680.
   The application of classic clinical manifestations correctly identified the drug or class causing intoxication in overdosed patients.

Olkkola K. Effect of charcoal–drug ratio on antidotal efficacy of oral activated charcoal in man. *Br J Clin Pharmacol* 1985;19:767–773.
   This in vitro *study demonstrated the effective drug:charcoal ratio to be 1:10 by weight.*

Pond SM, Lewis-Driver DJ, Williams G, et al. Gastric emptying in acute overdose: a prospective randomized controlled trial. *Med J Aust* 1995;163:345–349.
   This study failed to demonstrate clinical benefit from gastric emptying in all overdosed patients. However, when severity of illness was controlled for, patients with gastric emptying benefited.

Smilkstein MJ, Steedle D, Kulig KW, et al. Magnesium levels after magnesium containing cathartics. *J Toxicol Clin Toxicol* 1988;26:51–65.
This study demonstrated increased serum magnesium concentrations in human volunteers with normal renal function who were administered magnesium cathartics in repeated fashion.

Tenenbein M, Cohen S, Sitar DS. Whole bowel irrigation as a decontamination procedure after acute drug overdose. *Arch Intern Med* 1987;147:905–907.
This human volunteer study demonstrated the effectiveness of WBI in decreasing drug absorption.

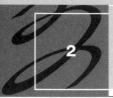

ACETAMINOPHEN
Steven B. Bird

I. BACKGROUND

A. Acetaminophen (APAP) is the most common drug involved in intentional and unintentional overdoses in the United States.

B. It is an active ingredient in hundreds of products, including combinations with opioid analgesics, antihistamines, and decongestants.

II. PATHOPHYSIOLOGY

A. In therapeutic doses, approximately 90% of APAP is metabolized by hepatic conjugation with sulfate or glucuronide to form inactive metabolites. A small portion is excreted unchanged in the urine.

B. The remaining fraction undergoes oxidation by the cytochrome P-450 mixed-function oxidases (CYP2E1) to yield the toxic intermediate NAPQI (N-acetyl-para-benzoquinoneimine), which then reacts with reduced glutathione (GSH) to form inactive products that are excreted in the urine.

C. NAPQI is a highly reactive electrophile that destroys both hepatocytes (centrilobular necrosis) and renal tubular cells. After overdose, the conjugation pathway becomes saturated, increasing the amount of APAP metabolized by the P-450 enzymes. GSH can then become depleted, allowing NAPQI to produce hepatotoxicity.

D. A single ingestion of more than 7.5 g in adults and more than 150 mg/kg in children should be considered potentially toxic. Toxicity can also occur after repeated ingestions of therapeutic or slightly greater doses of APAP, especially in persons who have conditions associated with increased cytochrome P-450 activity (chronic alcoholics) or glutathione depletion (malnutrition or acute illness).

III. DIAGNOSIS

A. Acute APAP toxicity can be divided into four phases based on the time after ingestion.

1. Stage 1 (0.5 to 24 hours). Patients may be asymptomatic or may be experiencing nausea, vomiting, and malaise.

2. Stage 2 (24 to 48 hours).

a. Patients have symptoms of hepatitis, including right upper quadrant abdominal pain, nausea, fatigue, and malaise.

    b. Elevation of aminotransferase levels usually occurs between 24 and 36 hours after ingestion but in severe cases can occur by 16 hours.

    c. Complications during stage 2 are related to the degree of liver and renal injury.

3. Stage 3 (72 to 96 hours).

    a. Liver injury becomes most pronounced, resulting in prolonged prothrombin time, elevated bilirubin, marked elevation of aminotransferases (>1,000 IU/L), metabolic acidosis, and hypoglycemia.

    b. Clinical symptoms reflect the degree of hepatic failure and encephalopathy. Oliguric or anuric renal failure can result from renal tubular necrosis. Pancreatitis and myocardial necrosis have also been reported.

    c. Most patients go on to full recovery, even those with markedly elevated aminotransferase levels. Death can occur 3 to 7 days after ingestion as a result of intractable metabolic disturbances, cerebral edema, or coagulopathy.

4. Stage 4 (4 days to 2 weeks).

    a. Patients who recover regain normal liver function. Recovery is often complete in 5 to 7 days in patients with minimal toxicity but can take 2 weeks or more in patients with more serious toxicity.

    b. No known cases have been seen of chronic or persistent liver abnormalities from APAP poisoning.

B. Laboratory studies. Obtain a serum APAP concentration between 4 and 24 hours after an acute, single ingestion.

    1. If the level falls on or above the treatment line on the Rumack–Matthew nomogram, the patient should be considered at risk for hepatotoxicity (Fig. 2-1).

    2. A single APAP concentration within 4 to 24 hours after ingestion should be sufficient to plan appropriate therapy, except in selected situations:

        a. If the time of ingestion is unknown and continued APAP absorption is a concern.

        b. If an extended-release formulation is suspected. In this case, a second APAP concentration should be obtained 4 to 6 hours after the initial one.

    3. If a patient is found to be at risk for toxicity, a complete blood count, electrolytes, blood urea nitrogen (BUN), creatinine, glucose, prothrombin and international normalized ratio (INR) times, aminotransferase levels, and bilirubin level should be obtained at admission and repeated every 24 hours until toxicity has resolved or been excluded.

IV. TREATMENT

A. Gastrointestinal (GI) Decontamination

    1. Actvated charcoal (see Chapter 1) should be administered for recent acute overdoses.

    2. Although charcoal can decrease the enteral absorption of the antidote N-acetylcysteine (NAC), this effect is clinically insignificant.

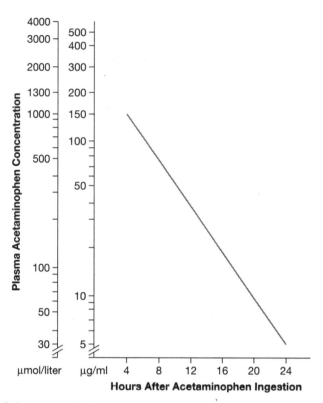

Figure 2-1. Rumack-Matthew acetaminophen treatment nomogram. Patients with acetaminophen concentrations on or above the line require treatment with *N*-acetylcysteine.

B. Antidotal Therapy

1. The specific antidote for APAP toxicity is NAC. Although several mechanisms explain its benefit in preventing APAP-induced liver and renal injury, it primarily acts as a glutathione precursor and substitute.

2. Begin NAC therapy after an acute overdose if the serum APAP concentration is in the toxic range on the nomogram, if the ingested amount is potentially toxic and more than 8 hours have elapsed since ingestion, or if serum aminotransferase levels are elevated and the patient has a history of APAP ingestion. In the latter two instances, NAC can be continued or discontinued when the APAP concentration becomes available.

3. The 72-hour oral treatment regimen consists of NAC (Mucomyst) given as a 140 mg/kg loading dose followed by 17 doses of 70 mg/kg every 4 hours. The 20% NAC solution should be diluted at least 3:1 with a carbonated or fruit beverage to improve palatability.

4. Aggressive antiemetic therapy may be needed to treat APAP- or NAC-induced vomiting. Metoclopramide, droperidol, or ondansetron can be

effective. NAC can also be given by a slow, continuous infusion through a gastric or duodenal tube. If vomiting occurs within 1 hour of any dose, that dose should be repeated.

5. A 20-hour intravenous NAC (Acetadote™) treatment protocol was recently approved for use in the United States.

C. Special Considerations

1. Late NAC administration (>24 hours after overdose) has shown clinical benefit in patients with APAP-induced fulminant liver failure.

2. Pregnant women should be treated according to standard guidelines regardless of gestational age of the fetus.

3. The nomogram has no validity in chronic APAP overdose. Patients with elevated APAP levels and no hepatotoxicity can be treated with NAC until the APAP is negligible. Patients who develop hepatotoxicity should be given a full course of NAC.

D. Liver Transplantation

1. Liver transplantation can be lifesaving in patients with severe liver failure.

2. Clinical criteria that predict mortality and hence the need for liver transplantation include

a. pH <7.30 after fluid resuscitation

b. Serum creatinine >3.4

c. Prothrombin time >100 sec (INR >6.5)

d. Grade III/IV encephalopathy

V. COMPLICATIONS. If the patient survives, complete recovery of hepatic function can be expected.

Selected Readings

Cetaruk EW, Dart RC, Hurlbut KM, et al. Tylenol Extended Relief overdose. *Ann Emerg Med* 1997;30:104–108.
Case series of patients with overdoses of extended-release preparations of acetaminophen (APAP) who demonstrated peak levels after 4 hours, suggesting the need for another APAP concentration 4 to 6 hours after the first.

Harrison PM, Wendon JA, Gimson AE, et al. Improvement by acetylcysteine of hemodynamics and oxygen transport in fulminant hepatic failure. *N Engl J Med* 1991;324:1852–1857.
Study of patients with acetaminophen-induced fulminant hepatic failure who demonstrated increases in oxygen delivery and consumption in response to acetylcysteine, perhaps accounting for its beneficial effect on survival in these patients.

Kao LW, Kirk MA, Furbee RB, et al. What is the rate of adverse events after oral N-acetylcysteine administered by the intravenous route to patients with suspected acetaminophen poisoning? *Ann Emerg Med* 2003;6:741–750.
Recommended procedure and case series reporting the indications and adverse events associated with administration of the oral N-acetylcysteine preparation by the intravenous route.

Keays R, Harrison PM, Wendon JA, et al. Intravenous acetylcysteine in paracetamol induced fulminant hepatic failure: a prospective controlled trial. *BMJ* 1991;303:1026–1029.

A controlled trial of patients with paracetamol-induced fulminant hepatic failure demonstrating decreased cerebral edema and increased survival in patients receiving intravenous N-acetylcysteine therapy comparedwith those who did not.

Mitchell JR, Thorgeirsson SS, Potter WZ, et al. Acetaminophen-induced hepatic injury: protective role of glutathione in man and rationale for therapy. *Clin Pharmacol Ther* 1974;16:676–684.
An animal study demonstrating that glutathione-like nucleophiles protect hepatocytes from injury caused by the reactive acetaminophen metabolite.

Renzi FP, Donovan JW, Martin TG, et al. Concomitant use of activated charcoal and N-acetylcysteine. *Ann Emerg Med* 1985;14:568–572.
A human volunteer study showing no difference in N-acetylcysteine levels after oral consumption between subjects who received charcoal and those who did not.

Rumack BH, Matthew H. Acetaminophen poisoning and toxicity. *Pediatrics* 1975; 55:871–876.
One of the first reviews to describe the toxicology of acetaminophen and proposals for treatment.

Rumack BH, Peterson RC, Koch GG, et al. Acetaminophen overdose: 662 cases with evaluation of oral acetylcysteine treatment. *Arch Intern Med* 1981;141:380–385.
One of the first and largest patient series to demonstrate the effectiveness of oral N-acetylcysteine treatment and the use of a nomogram to predict toxicity.

Smilkstein MJ, Knapp GL, Kulig KW, et al. Efficacy of oral N-acetylcysteine in the treatment of acetaminophen overdose: analysis of the National Multicenter Sudy (1976–1985). *N Engl J Med.* 1988;319:1557–1562.
Outcome study of more than 2,000 patients with acetaminophen poisoning treated with oral N-acetylcysteine, demonstrating a time-dependent relationship for its maximal efficacy.

Whitcomb DC, Block GD. Association of acetaminophen hepatotoxicity with fasting and ethanol use. *JAMA.* 1994;272:1845–1850.
A retrospective case series of patients, suggesting that acetaminophen hepatotoxicity appears to be enhanced by fasting and alcohol ingestion.

ALCOHOLS AND GLYCOLS

Steven B. Bird

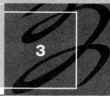

I. BACKGROUND

A. Ethanol (grain or beverage alcohol), methanol (wood alcohol), isopropanol (isopropyl or rubbing alcohol), and ethylene glycol are central nervous system (CNS) depressants.

B. CNS depressant potency increases as the carbon atom chain length increases.

II. PATHOPHYSIOLOGY

A. Ketoacidosis and hypoglycemia are caused by the hormonal, nutritional, metabolic, and intravascular volume changes caused by the consumption of ethanol and other alcohols.

B. The formation of toxic metabolites by hepatic alcohol dehydrogenase (ADH) is responsible for the renal toxicity of ethylene glycol, the ocular toxicity of methanol, and the increased anion gap metabolic acidosis (AGMA) caused by both.

C. The most common sources of methanol and ethylene glycol are automotive windshield washer fluid, gasoline antifreeze, and radiator antifreeze.

III. DIAGNOSIS

A. Clinical Presentation

1. Ethanol

    a. Patients with acute ethanol intoxication present with varying degrees of altered consciousness, including agitation, slurred speech, ataxia, stupor, and coma.

    b. Death from respiratory depression, aspiration, or cardiovascular collapse can occur in severe poisoning.

2. Isopropyl alcohol

    a. Isopropanol produces an ethanol-like intoxication.

    b. Symptoms of gastritis (e.g., abdominal pain, nausea, vomiting, possibly hematemesis) may also be present.

    c. Its acetone metabolite causes a spurious increase in serum creatinine. Therefore, an elevated creatinine level with normal blood urea nitrogen (BUN) can be a clue to the diagnosis.

3. Alcoholic ketoacidosis and hypoglycemia
   a. Patients with alcoholic ketoacidosis usually present with a recent history of binge drinking, poor nutritional intake, vomiting, and little or no measurable ethanol in their blood.
   b. Laboratory findings include mild to moderate AGMA and mild ketonemia. Dehydration is invariably present.
   c. Signs and symptoms of ethanol withdrawal may be present.
   d. Hypoglycemia causes an altered mental status ranging from agitation to confusion and coma.
   e. Symptoms of increased sympathetic activity caused by catecholamine release (e.g., diaphoresis and tachycardia) can also be present.
4. Ethylene glycol and methanol
   a. Because of their low molecular weight, high levels of an alcohol or ethylene glycol increase the serum osmolality. Hence, an elevated serum osmolality or osmolal gap (see Chapter 1) is a clue to their presence.
   b. Ethylene glycol and methanol poisoning should be suspected in all patients with a history of ingesting alcohol substitutes or in those who have an unexplained AGMA.
   c. Initially, an ethanol-like intoxication along with nausea, vomiting, and occasionally seizures dominates the clinical picture.
   d. Renal failure is a common sequela of ethylene glycol poisoning. Calcium oxalate crystalluria may be present. Cardiopulmonary effects (e.g, tachypnea, cyanosis, cardiogenic or noncardiogenic pulmonary edema) can occur in severe cases.
   e. In methanol toxicity, neurologic, ophthalmologic, and gastrointestinal symptoms predominate. Patients are frequently alert on admission and complain of headache and dizziness.
      (1) Visual symptoms are usually experienced acutely when the serum pH drops below 7.2.
      (2) Blurred vision, photophobia, scotomata, eye pain, partial or complete loss of vision, and visual hallucinations (e.g., bright lights, "snowstorm") have been reported.
      (3) Methanol can produce hemorrhagic gastritis and pancreatitis, resulting in abdominal pain, nausea, vomiting, and diarrhea.

B. Evaluation

1. Patients with a history of ethanol ingestion and mild to moderate intoxication need only determination of serum ethanol level and a fingerstick blood sugar evaluation. Those with severe intoxication or an unreliable history should be tested for levels of electrolytes, BUN, creatinine, glucose, complete blood count, arterial blood gas, ethanol, magnesium, calcium, and phosphorus as well as have liver function tests, prothrombin time determined, an electrocardiogram, a chest radiograph, and urinalysis.
2. Evaluation of known or suspected isopropanol poisoning should also include serum isopropanol and acetone serum levels.
3. Evaluation of known or suspected ethylene glycol and methanol poisoning should include quantitative serum levels of these compounds.
4. Microscopic examination of the urine for crystals should be performed if ethylene glycol ingestion is suspected or possible.

IV. TREATMENT

A. General Measures
1. Initial treatment includes supportive measures such as airway management, intravenous (IV) fluids, and cardiac monitoring.
2. Gastric aspiration via a nasogastric tube should be considered in patients with severe poisoning and within a few hours of isopropanol, ethylene glycol, or methanol ingestion.
3. Activated charcoal (see Chapter 1) should be considered when coingestants are suspected.
4. IV naloxone (2 mg) and thiamine hydrochloride (100 mg) should also be considered.
5. If bedside glucose testing reveals hypoglycemia, IV dextrose (25 to 50 g) should be administered.

B. Alcoholic Ketoacidosis and Hypoglycemia
1. IV fluids, glucose, and thiamine should be given for dehydration and to reverse the ketogenic process.
2. Prolonged hospitalization and refeeding of malnourished patients may be required.
3. The IV bolus of dextrose should be followed by a high carbohydrate meal or an infusion of 10% dextrose in patients with hypoglycemia.

C. Ethylene Glycol and Methanol
1. Large doses of sodium bicarbonate may be required to treat metabolic acidosis.
2. Primary antidotal therapy is fomepizole (Antizole).
   a. Prevents formation of toxic metabolites by competitively inhibiting the enzyme ADH.
   b. Induces its own metabolism, and therefore the dose changes over time.
   c. Consult package insert for dosing during concomitant hemodialysis.
3. If fomepizole is not readily available, a continuous ethanol infusion (to a goal of a serum concentration of 100 to 150 mg/dL) may be administered temporarily. Methanol and ethylene glycol are then eliminated slowly through pulmonary and renal excretion.
4. Indications for antidotal therapy include:
   a. An ethylene glycol or methanol level greater than 20 mg/dL.
   b. Unexplained AGMA with a low lactate level.
   c. Visual disturbances.
   d. Calcium oxalate crystalluria.
   e. Unexplained coma with a high osmolar gap and low ethanol level.
5. Patients poisoned by ethylene glycol should receive pyridoxine (100 mg) and thiamine (100 mg) IV daily until ethylene glycol levels are unmeasurable and acidemia has cleared.
6. Patients with methanol poisoning should be given IV leucovorin (1 mg/kg; maximal dose 50 mg) every 4 hours for a total of six doses.

D. Hemodialysis
1. Effectively removes ethanol, isopropanol, ethylene glycol, and methanol and their toxic metabolites and can correct metabolic abnormalities.

    2. Should be considered in severe poisoning that is unresponsive to other measures and in patients with ethylene glycol or methanol levels greater than 100 mg/dL (particularly those treated with ethanol).

V. COMPLICATIONS

    A. Renal failure from ethylene glycol poisoning usually resolves after several weeks to several months but can be permanent.

    B. Blindness resulting from methanol may be irreversible.

Selected Readings

Adams SL, Mathews JJ, Flatherty JJ. Alcoholic ketoacidosis. *Ann Emerg Med* 1987;16:90–97.
  Case presentation and review of the clinical and laboratory features of alcoholic ketoacidosis.

Baud FJ, Galliot M, Astier A, et al. Treatment of ethylene glycol poisoning with intravenous 4-methylpyrazole. *NEJM* 1988;319:97–100.
  Case report of the clinical and kinetic data of ethylene glycol treated with intravenous 4-methylpyrazole.

Brent J, McMartin K, Phillips S, et al. Fomepizole for the treatment of methanol poisoning *N Engl J Med* 2001;344:424–429.
  Case series of the effective treatment of methanol toxicity with the alcohol dehydrogenase inhibitor 4-methylpyrazole.

Charness ME, Simon RP, Greenberg DA. Ethanol and the nervous system. *N Engl J Med* 1989;321:442–454.
  An important review of the neurologic complications associated with ethanol abuse: intoxication, withdrawal, Wernicke's encephalopathy, dementia, cerebellar degeneration, and central pontine myelinolysis.

Dethlefs R, Naraqi S. Ocular manifestations and complications of acute methyl alcohol intoxication. *Med J Aust* 1978;2:483–485.
  Clinical series of 24 men with methanol toxicity showing that the incidence of permanent ocular abnormalities correlated with metabolic acidosis.

Hoffman RS, Smilkstein MJ, Howland MA, et al. Osmol gaps revisited: normal values and limitations. *J Toxicol Clin Toxicol* 1993;31:81–93.
  A study of 321 adults to evaluate the limitation of the osmol gaps in adults that concluded that small osmol gaps should not be used to eliminate a toxic alcohol ingestion.

Hoffman RS, Goldfrank LR. Ethanol-associated metabolic disorders. *Emerg Med Clin North Am* 1989;7:943–961.
  An excellent review and discussion of the fluid, electrolytes, acid-base, glucose, and nutritional complications causes by elevated ethanol levels.

Jacobsen D, Hewlett TP, Webb R, et al. Ethylene glycol intoxication: evaluation of kinetics and crystalluria. *Am J Med* 1988;84:145–152.
  A review of the two types of calcium oxalate crystals that are formed in the metabolism of ethylene glycol.

Jacobsen D, McMartin KE. Methanol and ethylene glycol poisonings: mechanism of toxicity, clinical course, diagnosis and treatment. *Med Toxicol* 1986;1:309–334.
  A review article on methanol and ethylene glycol toxicity with an excellent discussion of the clinically and biochemically similar characteristics that both compounds share.

Kruse JA, Cadnapaphorochni P. The serum osmole gap. *J Crit Care* 1994;9:185–197.
An in-depth review article on the different clinical indications for the use of osmol gap. Includes a helpful discussion regarding the limitations of its use.

LaCouture PG, Wason S, Abrams A, et al. Acute isopropyl alcohol intoxication: diagnosis and management. *Am J Med* 1983;75:680–686.
A review article focusing on the clinical presentation and management of isopropyl toxicity. Includes a helpful discussion of the differences between common toxic alcohols.

Martensson E, Olofsson U, Heath A. Clinical and metabolic features of ethanol–methanol poisoning in chronic alcoholics. *Lancet* 1988;1:327–328.
A study of 84 chronic alcoholic patients who ingested an ethanol–methanol suggesting that treatment should be based on the clinical presentation and acidosis and not solely on methanol blood concentrations.

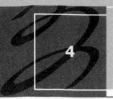

ANTIARRHYTHMIC AGENTS
D. Eric Brush

I. BACKGROUND

A. Antiarrhythmic drugs are classified on the basis of their physiologic effects and mechanisms of action (Table 4-1).

B. Class I agents are subdivided into groups IA, IB, and IC (Table 4-2).

C. Class II agents (β-blockers) and class IV agents (calcium channel blockers) are discussed in detail in separate chapters.

II. PATHOPHYSIOLOGY

A. Effects on Automaticity

1. The spontaneous depolarization (automaticity) of pacemaker myocytes in the sinoatrial (SA) and atrioventricular (AV) nodes is relatively insensitive to antiarrhythmic drugs but may be affected in states of high vagal tone or myocardial infarction.

2. Purkinje fibers produce escape beats in the context of AV nodal block.

3. Class I agents block automaticity in Purkinje fibers.

B. Effects on Intraventricular Conduction

1. Reentrant or circuit arrhythmias depend on slow conduction velocity to allow downstream tissues to recover from their refractory period.

2. Faster conduction results in the action potential reaching downstream tissue during the refractory phase, thereby preventing continuation of the circuit.

3. Slowing of conduction may explain some of the proarrhythmic nature of antiarrhythmic drugs.

4. Preferential slowing of conduction to zero in ischemic tissue may explain the antiarrhythmic effect of class IB drugs and amiodarone.

C. Effects on the Refractory Period

1. Most antiarrhythmic drugs prolong the refractory period, thereby decreasing the chance of a reentrant phenomenon.

2. Class IB drugs shorten the refractory period, which may explain drug-associated arrhythmogenesis in patients with reentrant tachycardia.

D. Effects on Early Afterdepolarizations (EADs)

1. Marked slowing of repolarization may trigger additional concurrent action potentials known as EADs.

TABLE 4-1   Vaughan–Williams Classification of Antiarrhythmic Actions

Class	Drugs	Actions
I	Quinidine Procainamide Disopyramide Moricizine Lidocaine Tocainide Mexiletine Flecainide Propafenone	Block fast sodium current (hence slow conduction)
II	Beta-blockers	Block effects of catecholamines
III	Amiodarone Sotalol Ibutilide Bretylium	Prolong action potential and, hence, refractoriness by blocking K^+ current
IV	Verapamil Diltiazem	Block cardiac calcium channel

Source: Irwin RS, Rippe JM. *Irwin and Rippe's Intensive Care Medicine,* 5th ed. Philadelphia: Lippincott Williams & Wilkins, 2003:1512.

TABLE 4-2   Subgroups of Class I Drugs

Class	Drugs	Effects on action potential	Summary of clinical effects
IA	Quinidine Procainamide Disopyramide Moricizine	Reduce rate of depolarization; prolong duration of action potential	Moderate slowing of cardiac conduction; prolongation of refractory periods
IB	Lidocaine Mexiletine Tocainide	Reduce rate of depolarization selectively in ischemic cells; shorten action potential duration	Selective depression of ischemic tissue; may shorten refractory periods
IC	Flecainide Propafenone	Marked depression of depolarization rate	Marked slowing of cardiac conduction; small increase in refractory periods

Source: Irwin RS, Rippe JM. *Irwin and Rippe's Intensive Care Medicine,* 5th ed. Philadelphia: Lippincott Williams & Wilkins, 2003:1513.

2. EADs may be responsible for induction of torsades de pointes (TdP).
3. Class IA and III agents can cause EADs and TdP, but class IB and IC agents do not.

III. DIAGNOSIS

A. Clinical Features and Manifestations

1. In chronic therapeutic dosing, toxicity may be precipitated by decreasing or increasing the dose of antiarrhythmic agents, concurrent use of other antiarrhythmic drugs (including digoxin), drug–drug metabolic interactions, hypoxia, acidosis, myocardial ischemia, hypokalemia, or hypomagnesemia.

2. Intentional overdose of any antiarrhythmic drug can cause acute toxicity.

3. Manifestations of poisoning include bradycardia, QRS and QTc prolongation, SA and AV nodal block, ventricular arrhythmias, and myocardial and respiratory depression culminating in intractable arrhythmias, cardiogenic shock, or death.

4. Features specific to individual agents include the following:

   a. Class IA agents
      (1) Prolonged QT interval with increased QRS and JT intervals.
      (2) Quinidine toxicity can result in cinchonism (headache, tinnitus, deafness, diplopia, confusion), vertigo, visual disturbances (blurred vision, photophobia, scotomata, contracted visual fields, yellow vision), or delirium. Severe toxicity causes coma, respiratory depression, seizures, vomiting, diarrhea, or cardiovascular collapse. α-Adrenergic blockade leads to hypotension.
      (3) Procainamide causes toxicity similar to quinidine but without α-adrenergic blockade. The active metabolite N-acetylprocainamide (NAPA) has class III effects and may accumulate in patients with renal failure leading to TdP. Of long-term users 40% develop a lupuslike syndrome that usually resolves with drug cessation.
      (4) Disopyramide toxicity is also similar to that of quinidine. Hypoglycemia has also been reported.

   b. Class IB agents
      (1) Usually have no effect on QRS or QT intervals.
      (2) Lidocaine toxicity usually results from dosing errors. Neurologic symptoms precede cardiac toxicity and include seizures, auditory disturbances, visual disturbances, paresthesias, ataxia, and respiratory arrest. QRS prolongation, AV block, bradycardia, and asystole characterize the cardiac effects.
      (3) Adverse effects of tocainide include nausea, vomiting, dizziness, paresthesias, tremor, ataxia, confusion, pulmonary fibrosis (0.1%), and agranulocytosis (0.2%). Massive overdose causes cardiovascular toxicity similar to that from lidocaine.
      (4) Mexiletine is structurally and clinically similar to lidocaine. Its longer half-life may cause prolonged seizures.

    c. Class IC agents
        (1) Increased QRS and QT (but not JT) intervals.
        (2) In therapeutic dosing, flecainide can worsen congestive heart failure (CHF) through negative inotropy. Other dose-related effects include blurred vision, dizziness, headache, nausea, and paresthesias. Overdose may cause QRS prolongation with a normal JT interval, bradycardia, hypotension, coma, and, less commonly, tachycardia and seizures.
        (3) Propafenone overdose is similar to that seen with flecainide.
    d. Class III agents
        (1) Increased JT and QT (but not QRS) intervals.
        (2) Amiodarone toxicity in chronic therapy includes pulmonary fibrosis (5% to 15%), sinus bradycardia, peripheral neuropathies, tremor, nervousness, corneal microdeposits, photosensitive dermatitis, and blue-grey skin. Toxicity from acute overdose may include ventricular tachycardia (VT), increased QT interval, or bradycardia.
        (3) Bretylium overdose results in initial sympathomimetic effects followed shortly by manifestations of adrenergic blockade. Postural hypotension is common.
        (4) Limited overdose information is available for ibutilide and dofetilide, but TdP is a concern.

B. Laboratory Studies
    1. Serum electrolytes, magnesium, and calcium may reveal derangements that can contribute to arrhythmias.
    2. With tocainide therapy, white blood cell counts should be monitored for agranulocytosis.
    3. Serum procainamide and NAPA levels should be monitored in the setting of worsening CHF or renal failure.
    4. Serum lidocaine level should be checked in patients on a drip for longer than 24 hours.
    5. Antiarrhythmic drug concentrations should be obtained if there is clinical evidence or suspicion of toxicity.

IV. TREATMENT

    A. The management of antiarrhythmic poisoning and overdose is summarized in Table 4-3 and includes:
        1. Cardiac monitoring, intravenous (IV) access, and a 12-lead ECG in all patients with potential poisoning.
        2. Treatment of underlying hypoxia, acidosis, myocardial ischemia, hypokalemia, or hypomagnesemia.
        3. Administration of activated charcoal (see Chapter 1) for recent acute overdose.
        4. Consideration of whole bowel irrigation (see Chapter 1) for patients with acute overdose of a sustained-release preparation.
        5. Initial treatment of hypotension with IV saline. Give small boluses to patients with heart failure. If no response after 2 L, administer

TABLE 4-3	Management of Life-Threatening Antiarrhythmic Drug Overdose

Supportive care
  Activated charcoal for all acute oral ingestions
  Correct acidosis, hypoxia
  Benzodiazepines for seizure control
Enhance drug elimination
  Activated charcoal
  Consider hemodialysis if appropriate
Hypotension
  Fluid administration
  Alkalinization (hypertonic $NaHCO_3$) for class I drugs
  Inotropes, vasopressors
  Pulmonary artery catheter for monitoring
  Circulatory assist devices
Impaired conduction
  Temporary pacing for atrioventricular block or bradycardia
  Alkalinization (hypertonic $NaHCO_3$) for class I drugs
Ventricular arrhythmias
  Torsades de pointes
    Temporary pacing
    $MgSO_4$
    Isoproterenol
  Monomorphic ventricular tachycardia
    Cardioversion, if causing hypotension
    Hypertonic $NaHCO_3$ for class I drugs
    Lidocaine, except for class IB drugs
    Overdrive pacing

Source: Irwin RS, Rippe JM. *Irwin and Rippe's Intensive Care Medicine,* 5th ed. Philadelphia: Lippincott Williams & Wilkins, 2003:1515.

vasopressors (see Chapter 1). Use of an intraaortic balloon pump (IABP) and partial cardiac bypass have been used successfully for the treatment of refractory hypotension.

6. IV sodium bicarbonate (NaHCO3), 1 mEq/kg (up to 50 mEq) bolus, and/or a drip of 150 mEq per liter of D5W at 1.5 times standard maintenance fluid rate based on weight for patients with prolonged QRS (>100 msec) or VT from class IA and IC agents. Titrate to serum pH of 7.45 to 7.55. Serum pH must be tested frequently to avoid excessive alkalemia. Check serum K^+ frequently.

7. Avoidance of class IA or IC agents for the treatment of antiarrhythmic-induced VT. Lidocaine may be considered because it does not depress conduction in normal tissue; however, it is often ineffective. Electrical cardioversion may be necessary for VT with cardiovascular instability.

8. Administration of IV magnesium sulfate (1 to 2 g over 5 to 10 min) for prolonged QT and TdP. Overdrive pacing, electrical cardioversion, or isoproterenol infusion can also be used.

9. Hemoperfusion utilizing a charcoal resin cartridge for refractory or prolonged disopyramide or NAPA toxicity. Hemodialysis is of limited utility given the large volume of distribution and high protein binding of antiarrhythmic drugs

Selected Readings

Braden GL, Fitzgibbons JP, Germain MJ, et al. Hemoperfusion for treatment of N-acetyl procainamide intoxication. *Ann Intern Med* 1986;105:64–65.
This is a case report describing the utilization of hemoperfusion in the context of NAPA toxicity.

Katz AM. Cardiac ion channels. *N Engl J Med* 1993;328:1244–1251.
This is a review article discussing the basic molecular physiology of cardiac ion channels providing a context for the mechanism of antiarhythmic pharmacology.

Kolecki PF, Curry SC. Poisoning by sodium channel blocking agents. *Crit Care Clin* 1997;Oct;13:829–848.
This review article summarizes the pathophysiology of sodium channel blocking toxicity and discusses treatment.

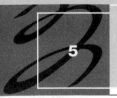

ANTICHOLINERGIC POISONING
Ivan E. Liang

I. BACKGROUND

A. Anticholinergic poisoning can be precipitated by a variety of agents including over-the-counter antihistamines, cough and cold preparations, sleep aids, prescription medications, plants, and mushrooms (Table 5-1)

B. It is manifested by a consistent and recognizable constellation of signs and symptoms—the anticholinergic toxidrome (Table 5-2).

C. Although most cases result in only mild toxicity, the potential exists for serious and life-threatening toxicity.

II. PATHOPHYSIOLOGY

A. Anticholinergic compounds antagonize the effects of the endogenous neurotransmitter acetylcholine (ACh).

B. Two types of ACh receptors—muscarinic and nicotinic—are distributed in the central nervous system (CNS), autonomic nervous system, and peripheral nervous system.

C. Anticholinergic agents primarily block muscarinic cholinergic receptors.

III. DIAGNOSIS

A. Clinical Manifestations

1. The anticholinergic toxidrome has been classically described by the mnemonic "Blind as a bat, dry as a bone, hot as Hades, red as a beet, and mad as a hatter."

2. The most common clinical findings include sinus tachycardia, mild hyperthermia, dry mucous membranes, dry and flushed skin, mydriasis, hypertension, urinary retention, and paralytic ileus. These symptoms can typically be expected to appear within 1 to 2 hours postingestion.

3. Other symptoms of CNS toxicity are somnolence, disorientation, hallucinations, mumbling speech, and a characteristic preoccupation with picking at nearby items.

4. The most serious manifestations include agitated delirium, hyperthermia, seizures, coma, and respiratory failure.

5. The clinical presentation can be complicated by other pharmacologic actions of the ingested agent (tricyclic antidepressants) or the actions of coingestants (acetaminophen, salicylates, sympathomimetics).

TABLE 5-1	Some Agents That Cause Anticholinergic Syndrome[a]

Pharmaceuticals

Antihistamines (H$_1$-blockers)
  Brompheniramine
  Chlorpheniramine
  Clemastine
  Cyclizine
  Cyproheptadine
  Dimenhydrinate
  Diphenhydramine
  Hydroxyzine
  Meclizine
  Pyrilamine
  Promethazine
  Tripelennamine
Antiparkinsonian drugs
  Benztropine
  Biperiden
  Ethopropazine
  Procyclidine
  Trihexyphenidyl
Antipsychotics
  Acetophenazine
  Chlorpromazine
  Fluphenazine
  Haloperidol
  Loxapine
  Molindone
  Olanzapine
  Perphenazine
  Prochlorperazine
  Quetiapine
  Risperidone
  Thioridazine
  Thiothixene
  Trifluoperazine

Antispasmodics
  Anisotropine
  Clidinium
  Dicyclomine
  Isometheptene
  Methantheline
  Propantheline
  Stramonium
  Tridihexethyl
Belladonna alkaloids and
    related synthetic congeners
  Atropine (racemic hyoscyamine)
  Glycopyrrolate
  Hyoscine
  Ipratropium
  Methscopolamine
  Scopolamine
Cyclic antidepressants
  Amitriptyline
  Amoxapine
  Desipramine
  Doxepin
  Imipramine
  Maprotiline
  Nortriptyline
  Protriptyline
  Trimipramine
  Zimelidine
Muscle relaxants
  Cyclobenzaprine
  Orphenadrine
Mydriatics
  Cyclopentolate
  Homatropine
  Tropicamide

Plants

Atropa belladonna (deadly nightshade)
Brugmansia arborea (angel's trumpet)
Brugmansia suaveolens (angel's trumpet)
Cestrum diurnum (day-blooming jessamine)
Cestrum nocturnum (night-blooming jessamine)

Cestrum parqui (willow-leaved jessamine)
Datura metel (downy thorn apple)
Datura stramonium (jimson weed)
Hyoscyamus niger (black henbane)
Lantana camara (wild sage)

[a]Many of these agents have other significant toxic manifestations in addition to their anticholinergic effects.

(*continued*)

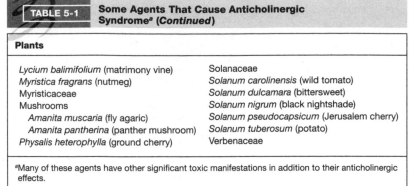

TABLE 5-1	Some Agents That Cause Anticholinergic Syndrome[a] (*Continued*)

Plants

Lycium balimifolium (matrimony vine)
Myristica fragrans (nutmeg)
Myristicaceae
Mushrooms
    Amanita muscaria (fly agaric)
    Amanita pantherina (panther mushroom)
Physalis heterophylla (ground cherry)

Solanaceae
Solanum carolinensis (wild tomato)
Solanum dulcamara (bittersweet)
Solanum nigrum (black nightshade)
Solanum pseudocapsicum (Jerusalem cherry)
Solanum tuberosum (potato)
Verbenaceae

[a]Many of these agents have other significant toxic manifestations in addition to their anticholinergic effects.

Source: Irwin RS, Rippe JM. *Irwin and Rippe's Intensive Care Medicine,* 5th ed. Philadelphia: Lippincott Williams & Wilkins, 2003:1381.

TABLE 5-2	Manifestations of the Anticholinergic Syndrome

Peripheral anticholinergic signs and symptoms
    Cardiovascular: hypertension and tachycardia
    Skin: dry and flushed with dry mucous membranes
    Eyes: mydriasis (variable)
    Genitourinary: urinary retention and decreased bowel sounds (ileus)
Central anticholinergic signs and symptoms
    Loss of short-term memory and confusion, disorientation, psychomotor agitation
    Visual/auditory hallucinations or frank psychosis
    Incoordination and ataxia
    Picking or grasping movements and extrapyramidal reactions
    Seizures
    Coma with respiratory failure

Source: Irwin RS, Rippe JM. *Irwin and Rippe's Intensive Care Medicine,* 5th ed. Philadelphia: Lippincot Williams & Wilkins, 2003:1381.

B. Differential Diagnosis

1. Other toxic causes of physiological excitation include sympathomimetics, hallucinogens, and withdrawal syndromes (see Table 1-1), although sympathomimetic agents usually induce diaphoresis.

2. In contrast to anticholinergic poisoning, these agents and conditions are usually associated with pallor, diaphoresis, and increased bowel and bladder activity.

C. Ancillary Studies

1. Initial testing should include electrolytes, blood urea nitrogen (BUN), creatinine, glucose, creatine phosphokinase (to evaluate for rhabdomyolysis), and acetaminophen levels (frequent coingestant).

2. A 12-lead ECG should be obtained, with close attention paid to the QRS duration.
3. Specific drug levels are not generally useful. Qualitative toxicology tests may confirm the presence of an anticholinergic agent. Management is based on the history and clinical status of the patient.

IV. MANAGEMENT

A. Advanced life support measures should be instituted as necessary. All patients should have continuous cardiac monitoring and intravenous (IV) access established.

B. Activated charcoal should be considered in patients with oral exposures. Because of delayed gastric emptying and impaired gut motility, gastrointestinal decontamination may prove beneficial even several hours after ingestion. Repeated doses of charcoal should not be given in the setting of an ileus or obstruction because of the risk of impaction or aspiration.

C. Significant cardiovascular toxicity is rare. Tachycardia and hypertension rarely require specific therapy.

D. Patients with mild psychomotor hyperactivity can be observed or treated with nonspecific sedation with benzodiazepines. Phenothiazines, butyrophenones, and other agents with anticholinergic activity should be avoided.

E. Physostigmine, a specific antidote, is the treatment of choice for significant agitation and delirium, particularly if associated with rhabdomyolysis and hyperthermia. Benzodiazepines can also be used, but large doses are often required, resulting in CNS depression, an increased incidence of aspiration, and the need for endotracheal intubation.
1. Physostigmine is an acetylcholinesterase inhibitor that can reverse the anticholinergic toxicity by increasing synaptic acetylcholine peripherally and centrally.
2. Overdose of tricyclic antidepressants or other agents with sodium channel blocking activity is a relative contraindication to the use of physostigmine. Evidence of sodium channel blockade on electrocardiogram, such as QRS prolongation above 100 milliseconds or an R wave greater than the S wave in AVR, is an absolute contraindication.
3. The dose for adults is 1 to 2 mg, given as a slow IV infusion over 2 to 5 minutes. The pediatric dose is 0.02 mg/kg, up to 0.5 mg. Repeat doses can be given after 10 to 20 minutes if anticholinergic effects persist or recur.
4. Response is usually quick (within minutes) and remarkable, but recurrent toxicity is relatively common.
5. Administration of physostigmine carries a theoretical risk for cholinergic excess resulting in bradycardia, bronchorrhea and bronchospasm, and seizures. Such adverse effects can be treated with atropine.
6. Physostigmine will significantly potentiate depolarizing neuromuscular blockade agents such as succinylcholine.

F. Further interventions that may be indicated include bladder decompression by catheterization for urinary retention, aggressive cooling and neuromuscular paralysis for hyperthermia, benzodiazepines or phenobarbital for seizures, and correction of dehydration with IV fluids.

G. Patients with mild toxicity can be medically cleared if toxicity resolves after 6 to 8 hours of observation.

H. Patients presenting with progressive, moderate, or severe toxicity should be admitted to an intensive or intermediate care unit.

V. COMPLICATIONS

A. Anticholinergic effects usually resolve within 1 to 2 days as the offending agent is eliminated.

B. Recovery from secondary organ-system dysfunction resulting from complications such as pulmonary aspiration, rhabdomyolysis, and hyperthermia may take much longer.

Selected Readings

Brown JH, Taylor P. Muscarinic receptor agonists and antagonists. In: Hardman JG, Limbird LE, Gilman AG, eds. *Goodman and Gilman's the pharmacological basis of therapeutics*, 10th ed. New York: McGraw-Hill; 2001:155–174.
An overview of the pharmacology, adverse effects, and toxicity of antimuscarinic drugs.

Burns MJ, Linden CH, Graudins A, et al. A comparison of physostigmine and benzo-diazepines for the treatment of anticholinergic poisoning. *Ann Emerg Med* 2000;35(4):374–381.
This retrospective review found that physostigmine was more effective and associated with fewer complications than benzodiazepines for the treatment of anticholinergic agitation and delirium.

Schneir AB, Offerman SR, Ly BT, et al. Complications of diagnostic physostigmine administration to emergency department patients. *Ann Emerg Med* 2003;42(1): 14–19.
Two studies that review presentations of anticholinergic toxicity and use of physostigmine.

ANTICONVULSANTS
Ivan E. Liang

6

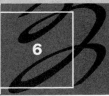

I. PHENYTOIN (diphenylhydantoin)

A. Background
1. Multiple formulations are available (intravenous [IV], oral, extended release, prodrug fosphenytoin).
2. Therapeutic serum levels are 10 to 20 µg/mL.

B. Pathophysiology
1. Phenytoin blocks sodium channels in excitable cell membranes and prevents seizure foci from discharging adjacent areas. It also has class IB antiarrhythmic activity (see Chapter 4).
2. Oral absorption is slow and erratic. Peak blood levels occur 2 to 9 hours after a therapeutic dose. Following overdose, absorption may continue for up to 7 days.
3. Elimination follows zero-order (saturation) kinetics. At therapeutic blood levels (10 to 20 µg/mL), the half-life is about 22 hours. At higher levels, the half-life is considerably longer.

C. Diagnosis
1. Phenytoin causes central nervous system (CNS) depression with cerebellar–vestibular dysfunction (ataxia, nystagmus, diplopia, opthalmoplegia).
2. Toxicity from chronic and acute exposure is similar and correlates with serum drug concentrations.
   a. Levels of 20 to 40 µg/mL are associated with nausea, normal to dilated pupils, nystagmus, blurred vision, diplopia, slurred speech, ataxia, tremor, and lethargy.
   b. Levels of 40 to 90 µg/mL are associated with increasing CNS depression, sluggish pupils, and decreased reflexes. Paradoxical excitation (agitation, hallucinations, seizures) sometimes occurs.
   c. Levels greater than 90 µg/mL are associated with coma and respiratory depression.
3. Cardiotoxicity from oral phenytoin is exceedingly rare. Arrhythmias (particularly bradycardia and atrioventricular [AV] block but also ventricular tachycardia and asystole), hypotension, congestive heart failure, and respiratory arrest have occurred with rapid (>50 mg/min) IV administration. These effects are primarily the result of propylene glycol (phenytoin vehicle) toxicity and generally spontaneously resolve with discontinuation of the infusion. Fosphenytoin is water soluble and much less likely to cause these effects.

4. Non–dose-dependent hypersensitivity reactions include fever, rash, eosinophilia, hepatitis, lymphadenopathy, myositis, vasculitis, rhabdomyolysis, and hemolytic anemia.

5. The differential diagnosis includes intoxication by other anticonvulsants, sedative hypnotics, neuroleptic agents, and other CNS depressants. Nontoxicologic causes of CNS depression and neurologic dysfunction such as stroke, infection, and trauma must be considered.

6. Evaluation should include complete blood count (CBC), electrolytes, blood urea nitrogen (BUN), creatinine, glucose, electrocardiogram, and serial serum phenytoin concentrations.

D. Management

1. Advanced life support measures and supportive care should be instituted as necessary (see Chapter 1). All patients with phenytoin intoxication or significant overdose should have IV access established. Because intoxication often progresses after oral overdose, frequent reevaluations are necessary.

2. Hypotension and arrhythmias during IV administration of phenytoin should be treated with immediate discontinuation of infusion. IV fluids should be given for persistent hypotension. Cardiac dysrhythmias should be treated according to usual protocols, but other Type IB antidysrhythmics (see Chapter 4) should be avoided.

3. Paradoxical seizures should be treated with benzodiazepines.

4. Activated charcoal (see Chapter 1) should be given for recent oral overdose.

5. Multidose activated charcoal (see Chapter 1) can increase phenytoin elimination and should be considered in patients with moderate to severe poisoning.

6. Whole bowel irrigation (see Chapter 1) should be considered if prolonged absorption continues despite appropriate gastrointestinal (GI) decontamination.

7. Patients with acute ingestions should be observed for at least 4 to 6 hours and have a repeat phenytoin level check 3 to 4 hours after the initial one. Minimal requirements for safe discharge should include:
   a. Serum drug concentrations that are decreasing.
   b. Clinical improvement (ambulatory and able to feed self).
   c. Psychiatric evaluation for patients with intentional ingestions.
   d. Reliable caregiver.

8. Patients with moderate, severe, or progressive clinical toxicity or symptoms should be admitted to a monitored unit.

E. Complications.
Phenytoin toxicity resolves as serum concentrations decrease unless complications, such as pulmonary aspiration and hypoxia, develop.

II. VALPROIC ACID

A. Background

1. Valproic acid (VPA) is available in multiple oral formulations. It can also be administered IV.

2. Therapeutic serum levels are 50 to 100 μg/mL.

B. Pathophysiology

1. VPA is thought to act by increasing CNS levels of γ-aminobutyric acid (GABA), perhaps with some direct effects on sodium and potassium channels in neurons.
2. Serum concentrations peak in 1 to 4 hours after immediate release, 4 to 5 hours after enteric-coated divalproex sodium, and up to 17 hours after overdose.
3. At therapeutic dosing, the elimination half-life averages 10.6 hours. After overdose it may extend to 30 hours.
4. VPA disrupts amino acid and fatty acid metabolism and can cause hyperammonemia, with or without hepatitis, at therapeutic doses.

C. Diagnosis

1. VPA overdose causes CNS depression without cerebellar–vestibular effects.
2. Vital signs are variable, usually with mild hypotension, mild tachycardia, decreased respiratory rate, and elevated or depressed temperature.
3. Ingestions of 200 mg/kg and serum concentrations of 180 μg/mL are associated with significant CNS depression.
4. VPA is an unmeasured anion and high drug levels can cause an increased anion gap metabolic acidosis.
5. Non–dose-dependent adverse effects include hepatitis, pancreatitis, anemia, neutropenia, and alopecia.
6. The differential diagnosis is the same as for phenytoin.
7. Evaluation should include CBC, electrolytes, BUN, creatinine, glucose, ammonia, liver function tests, ECG, and serial VPA levels.

D. Management

1. Supportive care, decontamination measures, and disposition considerations are the same as for phenytoin.
2. IV naloxone (see Chapter 30) can reverse VPA-induced CNS depression and should be considered in comatose patients. Efficacy is variable and inconsistent.
3. Hemodialysis and hemoperfusion are effective in reducing VPA concentrations and should be considered in patients with levels greater than 1,000 μm/mL or severe clinical toxicity.
4. L-Carnitine (50 mg/kg/day infusion or slow bolus; 50 to 100 mg/kg/day orally, divided into two or three doses, maximum 3 g/day) can be used for the treatment of hyperammonemia.

E. Complications are the same as for phenytoin.

III. CARBAMAZEPINE

A. Background

1. Carbamazepine (CBZ) is an oral medication that is structurally similar to phenytoin and tricyclic antidepressants.
2. Therapeutic serum levels are 4 to 12 mg/L.

B. Pathophysiology

   1. CBZ has multiple actions, including stabilization of sodium channels and alteration of neurotransmitter activity.
   2. Oral absorption of CBZ is erratic and inconsistent with unpredictable intermittent surges of absorption. Peak concentrations typically occur 6 to 24 hours postingestion.
   3. CBZ is metabolized by the liver cytochrome P-450 enzymes primarily to the active metabolite CBZ-epoxide. Enzyme autoinduction occurs. The half-life decreases from 18 to 55 hours to 5 to 26 hours with chronic use.
   4. Acute ingestion of more than 10 mg/kg is potentially toxic.

C. Diagnosis

   1. Symptoms of acute or chronic intoxication include:
   a. CNS depression with cerebellar–vestibular dysfunction (see Phenytoin).
   b. Anticholinergic manifestations (sinus tachycardia; mydriasis; red, flushed skin; dry mucous membranes; urinary retention; ileus; and hyperthermia; see Chapter 5).
   c. Movement disorders (dystonia, oculogyric crisis, choreoathetosis).
   d. Cardiotoxicity similar to that seen with tricyclic antidepressants (see Chapter 7) can occur but is rare.
   e. Although levels do not correlate well with clinical toxicity, severe toxicity is usually associated with levels over 40 mg/L. CBZ can cause a false-positive result for tricyclic antidepressants on drug screens.
   2. Non–dose-dependent adverse effects include bone marrow suppression, hepatitis, tubulointerstitial renal disease, cardiomyopathy, hyponatremia, and exfoliative dermatitis.
   3. Evaluation should include CBC, electrolytes, BUN, creatinine, glucose, ECG, and serial CBZ serum concentrations.

D. Management

   1. Supportive care, decontamination measures, and disposition considerations are the same as for phenytoin.
   2. Cardiotoxicity should be treated the same as with tricyclic antidepressants (see Chapter 7).
   3. Hemoperfusion can reduce CBZ concentrations, although its effectiveness does not appear superior to multidose activated charcoal. Hemodialysis is not useful.

E. Complications are the same as for phenytoin.

IV. OTHER ANTICONVULSANTS

A. Background

   1. There is little overdose information regarding other anticonvulsants, and treatment is almost exclusively supportive.
   2. GI decontamination is indicated for recent ingestions (see phenytoin).
   3. Serum drug levels are not readily available or clinically useful.
   4. Hemodialysis may be effective for enhancing gabapentin and topiramate elimination but is rarely necessary.

B. Gabapentin

1. Mechanism of action is unknown. Despite its name, it does not appear to act at the GABA receptor.
2. Peak serum levels occur 1 to 3 hours postingestion with a half-life of 5 to 7 hours.
3. Symptoms of toxicity include CNS depression, nystagmus, diplopia, unsteady gait, mood changes, and headache.
4. Toxicity typically resolves within 48 hours.

C. Lamotrigine

1. Mechanisms of action and toxicity are similar to those of phenytoin.
   a. Peak plasma levels occur 1 to 4 hours postingestion, with a half-life of 12 to 50 hours in therapeutic dosing.
   b. Tricyclic antidepressant–like cardiac effects have been observed and should be treated the same as for tricyclic antidepressants (see Chapter 7).
2. Non–dose-dependent adverse effects include Stevens–Johnson syndrome, toxic epidermal necrolysis, drowsiness, dizziness, headache, unsteady gait, tremor, diplopia, and nausea.

D. Felbamate

1. Appears to act via the $GABA_A$ receptor, similarly to sedative hypnotics (see Chapter 32).
2. Peak plasma levels occur 1 to 4 hours postingestion, with an elimination half-life of 20 to 23 hours.
3. Felbamate has significant effects on cytochrome P-450 enzymes. It induces metabolism of CBZ and inhibits metabolism of phenytoin and VPA.
4. Toxic effects include agitation/altered mental status, ataxia, nystagmus, weakness, and renal failure crystalluria (felbamate crystals).
5. Non–dose-dependent adverse effects include aplastic anemia and hepatic failure as well as nausea, vomiting, abdominal pains, headache, tachycardia, visual symptoms, tremors, and ataxia.

E. Topiramate

1. Mechanism of action is uncertain but may include sodium channel blockade or GABA effects.
2. Peak plasma levels occur at 1.8 to 4.3 hours, with an elimination half-life of 18 to 24 hours.
3. Toxicity primarily involves CNS depression.
4. Non–dose-dependent adverse effects include cognitive dysfunction, paresthesias, sedation, dizziness, fatigue, weight loss, diarrhea, and urolithiasis.

Selected Readings

Apfelbaum JD, Caravati EM, Kems WP, et al. Cardiovascular effects of carbamazepine toxicity. *Ann Emerg Med* 1995;25:631–635.
A retrospective review of 72 patients with carbamazepine overdose showing a low incidence of significant cardiovascular toxicity.

Chua HC, et al. Elimination of phenytoin in toxic overdose. *Clin Neurol Neurosurg* 2000;102(1):6–8.
Prospective pharmacokinetic study of phenytoin overdose, demonstrating linear elimination at a rate of 3.6 to 5.9 mg/L/day.

Eamest MP, Marx JA, Drury LR. Complications of intravenous phenytoin for acute treatment of seizures: Recommendations for usage. *JAMA* 1983;249:762–765.
Discussion of the potential complications of parenteral phenytoin administration. Guidelines are based on a prospective study of 200 patients.

O'Donnell J, Bateman DN. Lamotrigine overdose in an adult. *J Toxicol Clin Toxicol* 2000;38(6):659–660.
Reviews a 4.5 g ingestion resulting in ataxia and nystagmus.

Rengstorff DS, Milstone AP, Seger DL, et al. Felbamate overdose complicated by massive crystalluria and acute renal failure. *J Toxicol Clin Toxicol* 2000:38(6):667–669.
Large ingestion (peak serum level of 470 mg/L) with crystalluria that resolved with IV hydration.

Spiller, HA. Management of carbamazepine overdose. *Pediatr Emerg Care* 2001: 17(6):452–456.
Excellent overview.

Spiller HA,Krenzelok EP, Klein-Schwartz W, et al. Multicenter case series of valproic acid ingestion: serum concentrations and toxicity. *J Toxicol Clin Toxicol* 2000; 38(7):755–760. Erratum in *J Toxicol Clin Toxicol* 2001;39(1):115.
Large clinical and pharmacokinetic study; peak levels of greater than 450 mg/L were associated with worse outcomes, of greater than 850 mg/L with coma and acidosis.

Wyte CD, Berk WA. Severe oral phenytoin overdose does not cause cardiovascular morbidity. *Ann Emerg Med* 1991;20:508–512.
A retrospective review of severe phenytoin overdose showing no evidence of cardiovascular complications and no deaths.

ANTIDEPRESSANT POISONING
D. Eric Brush

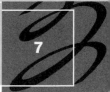

7

I. BACKGROUND

A. Antidepressants encompass a variety of drugs that have a cyclic component to their structure, including monoamine oxidase inhibitors (MAOIs) and selective serotonin reuptake inhibitors (SSRIs) (Table 7-1).

B. Toxic effects include central nervous system (CNS) and cardiovascular depression, arrhythmias, and seizures as well as MAOI drug and food interactions and the serotonin syndrome.

II. PATHOPHYSIOLOGY

A. Pharmacology

1. Tricyclic antidepressants inhibit the reuptake of norepinephrine, dopamine (DA), and serotonin (5-HT) in the CNS. Other effects include postsynaptic blockade of histamine, dopamine (DA), acetylcholine (ACh), 5-HT, norepinephrine, and γ-aminobutyric acid (GABA) receptors. Peripheral α-receptor blockade contributes to hypotension. Class IA antiarrhythmic effects (i.e., Na^+ channel blockade) (see Chapter 4) largely mediate the cardiac and neurologic toxicity.

2. Other cyclic agents inhibit the reuptake of 5-HT and have varying degrees of norepinephrine reuptake inhibition. Buproprion is unique in that its structure resembles that of amphetamine, which partly explains its propensity for causing seizures.

3. SSRIs inhibit the reuptake of 5-HT but have minimal effects on other neurotransmitters.

4. MAOIs inhibit MAO enzymes that degrade biogenic amines (E, norepinephrine, 5-HT, DA) in nerve terminals and the gut wall. This leads to increased catecholamine stores in nerve terminals that are released by indirect-acting sympathomimetics such as amphetamines, ephedrine, and tyramine. It also increases the bioavailability of ingested amines (sympathomimetic drugs and tyramine/tryptophan in food).

5. The serotonin syndrome results from excessive CNS serotonergic activity due to increased 5-HT production (e.g., from ingested tryptophan), increased presynaptic release (e.g., by sympathomimetics), reuptake inhibition (e.g., by cyclic and SSRI antidepressants), receptor agonism (e.g., by bromocryptine, L-dopa, lithium, and tryptans), and inhibited metabolism (e.g., by MAOIs).

TABLE 7-1	Antidepressants	
Monocyclic	Protriptyline	**MAOI**
Buproprion	Nortriptyline	Moclobemide
Bicyclic	**Tetracyclic**	Pargyline
Venlafaxine	Maprotiline	Phenelzine
Tricyclic	Mirtazapine	Tranylcypromine
Amitriptyline	**"Atypical" tetracyclic**	Isocarboxazid
Imipramine	Trazadone	**SSRI**
Doxepin	Nefazodone	Citalopram
Trimipramine	**Heterocyclic**	Escitalopram
Clomipramine	Loxapine	Fluoxetine
Desipramine	Amoxapine	Paroxetine
		Sertraline

B. Pharmacokinetics

1. Cyclic antidepressants are well absorbed orally, with peak serum concentrations occurring 2 to 6 hours after ingestion. Volume of distribution is large; protein binding is extensive. Metabolism is predominately hepatic. Many have active metabolites. Elimination half-life is variable and ranges from 8 to 30 hours. Absorption and elimination may be prolonged after overdose. Buproprion is available in a sustained-release formulation and can display significantly delayed peak serum concentrations causing delayed toxicity.

2. Although readily absorbed, maximal MAO inhibition may not occur until 2 to 3 weeks after beginning MAOI therapy. Maximal effects are also delayed after acute overdose. Because most MAOIs are irreversible inhibitors of MAO, inhibition of MAO activity may persist for 2 to 3 weeks after overdose or cessation of therapy (until new enzyme can be synthesized).

III. DIAGNOSIS

A. Clinical Manifestations

1. Monocyclic and heterocyclic antidepressants
   a. Can cause seizures as well as CNS depression.
      (1) Seizures resulting from bupropion are usually brief, may occur with therapeutic dosing and without any prodrome, and can be delayed up to 24 hours after overdose with sustained-release preparations.
      (2) Seizures resulting from amoxapine can be recurrent and prolonged, leading to rhabdomyolysis.
   b. Cardiotoxicity appears limited, although reports of conduction delay exist.
2. Bicyclic antidepressants
   a. Generally cause only mild tachycardia.
   b. Venlafaxine can cause seizures, QRS and QT widening, and ventricular dysrhythmias.

3. Tricyclic antidepressants

    a. Onset and progression of toxicity following tricyclic antidepressant overdose is rapid, beginning within 30 minutes and peaking within 2 to 6 hours.

    b. Early manifestations include tachycardia, mild hypertension, and other anticholinergic effects (see Chapter 5).

    c. Coma, seizures, hypotension, and dysrhythmias may ensue.

    d. ECG findings include intraventricular conduction delays, repolarization abnormalities, ventricular tachydysrhythmias, bradycardia, atrioventricular block, and asystole.

        (1) Sinus tachycardia is the earliest finding.

        (2) With increasing toxicity, slowing of conduction through the right bundle shifts the overall QRS axis rightward, causing a terminal 40 msec axis of 130 degrees to 270 degrees in the frontal plane. This is recognized as a widened S wave in leads I and aVL and an R wave in aVR.

        (3) The QRS, QT, and JT intervals also become prolonged.

        (4) Sinus tachycardia with aberrant conduction is often mistaken for ventricular tachycardia.

        (5) An R wave larger than 3 mm or greater than the S wave amplitude in AVR and a QRS of more than 0.16 second are associated with severe clinical toxicity.

        (6) JT (and hence QT) prolongation can occur with therapeutic doses.

    e. Anticholinergic effects may also become prominent during emergence from coma.

4. Tetracyclic antidepressants

    a. CNS and cardiovascular toxicity resulting from maprotiline is similar to that from tricyclic antidepressants.

    b. Less pronounced effects are seen with mirtazapine overdose.

5. "Atypical" tetracyclic antidepressants

    a. Overdose commonly causes tachycardia and CNS depression.

    b. QT prolongation and torsades de pointes (TdP) can occur.

6. MAOIs

    a. Acute overdose

        (1) Toxicity may not develop until 6 to 24 hours after ingestion and can last for several days.

        (2) Initial manifestations are the result of sympathetic hyperactivity and include agitation, confusion, tremor, and hyperreflexia-increased vital signs (BP, HR, RR, and T).

        (3) This may be followed by cardiovascular collapse as excitatory neurotransmitter stores become depleted.

        (4) Complications include rhabdomyolysis, electrolyte abnormalities, lactic acidosis, and multisystem organ failure.

    b. Drug and food interactions

        (1) Patients taking MAOIs who ingest indirect acting sympathomimetics (amphetamines, ephedrine, phenylephrine) or food high in tyramine (aged cheese, smoked and pickled meats, red wine, pasteurized light and pale beers) can rapidly (within 30 to 60 minutes) develop a "hypertensive crisis" with agitation, tachycardia, hyperthermia, and seizures.

(2) The duration of effect of all sympathomimetics may be prolonged, regardless of the route of administration.

7. Selective serotonin reuptake inhibitors

    a. Overdose in isolation generally results in mild CNS depression and tachycardia.

    b. Citalopram (and possibly escitalopram) can cause seizures, QT prolongation, and wide-complex tachycardia with doses greater than 600 mg.

8. Serotonin syndrome

    a. Can be caused by all antidepressants, alone or in combination, in therapeutic doses and overdose, or when combined with other serotonergic agents. It is most common during chronic therapy, when the dose is increased or another serotonergic agent is added.

    b. Manifestations include altered mental status, increased muscle activity (hyperreflexia, clonus), and autonomic findings (hypertension, hypotension, tachycardia, hyperthermia).

    c. The diagnosis is based on the history of drug exposure and examination findings (Table 7-2.)

B. Evaluation

1. All patients with antidepressant poisoning should have an electrocardiogram (ECG) as well as serum electrolytes, blood urea nitrogen (BUN), creatinine, and glucose testing.

2. Those with an abnormal ECG should also have serum Mg^{2+} and Ca^{2+} levels checked.

3. Those with significant CNS depression or seizures should have a chest x-ray and creatine phosphokinase (CPK) level tested.

4. Frequent clinical and ECG reevaluations should be performed.

5. Drug concentrations are not readily available and have no utility in the management of overdose.

6. False-positive urine immunoassay results for tricyclic antidepressants may be caused by carbamazepine, cyclobenzaprine, cyproheptadine diphenhydramine, prochlorperazine, perphenazine, quetiapine, or thioridazine.

TABLE 7-2   The Hunter Serotonin Toxicity Criteria: Decision Rules
In the presence of a serotonergic agent: 1. IF (spontaneous clonus = yes) THEN serotonin toxicity = YES 2. ELSE IF (inducible clonus = yes) AND [(agitation = yes) OR (diaphoresis = yes)] THEN serotonin toxicity = YES 3. ELSE IF (ocular clonus = yes) AND [(agitation = yes) OR (diaphoresis = yes)] THEN serotonin toxicity = YES 4. ELSE IF (tremor = yes) AND (hyperreflexia = yes) THEN serotonin toxicity = YES 5. ELSE IF (hypertonic = yes) AND (temperature >38°C) AND [(ocular clonus = yes) OR (inducible clonus = yes)] then serotonin toxicity = YES 6. ELSE serotonin toxicity = NO
Source: Dunkley EJ, Isbister GK, Sibbritt D, et al. The Hunter Serotonin Toxicity Criteria: simple and accurate diagnostic decision rules for serotonin toxicity. *Q J Med* 96:635–642, 2003.

III. TREATMENT

A. General Measures

1. All patients with potential poisoning should undergo cardiac monitoring and have intravenous (IV) access established.
2. Advanced life support measures should be instituted as necessary. Supportive measures should include treatment of underlying hypoxia, acidosis, hypokalemia, or hypomagnesemia.
3. Hypotension should initially be treated with IV saline. If the patient does not respond after 2 L, administer vasopressors (see Chapter 1). Intraaortic balloon pump (IABP) and partial cardiac bypass could be used for the treatment of refractory hypotension.
4. Seizures should be treated with benzodiazepines.
5. Activated charcoal (see Chapter 1) should be considered for recent acute overdose. For buproprion SR ingestion, whole bowel irrigation (see Chapter 1) should also be considered.

B. Cyclic Antidepressant Overdose

1. Patients with cyclic antidepressant overdose who remain or become asymptomatic and have a normal ECG may be discharged after 6 hours of observation.
2. Overdose with sustained-release buproprion is an exception and necessitates admission for 24 hours because of the potential for delayed seizures.
3. Patients who are symptomatic or show ECG changes should have cardiac monitoring and be observed until they return to normal.
4. Patients with coma, seizures, hypotension, or arrhythmias should be admitted to an intensive care unit (ICU).
5. Administer IV sodium bicarbonate to patients with tricyclic antidepressant overdose and QRS greater than 100 msec) or ventricular tachycardia (VT; see Chapter 4).
6. Avoid class IA or IC antiarrhythmics (see Chapter 4) for tricyclic antidepressant–induced VT. Lidocaine (class IB) may be considered because it does not depress conduction; however, it is often ineffective. Electrical cardioversion may be necessary for VT with cardiovascular instability.
7. Administer IV magnesium sulfate for prolonged QT and TdP (see Chapter 4). Overdrive pacing, electrical cardioversion, or isoproterenol infusion can also be used.
8. Physostigmine can be given for anticholinergic agitation and delirium (see Chapter 5), but it is contraindicated if tricyclic antidepressant effects are noted on ECG or if a period of observation has not excluded worsening toxicity.
9. Patients with tachycardia and hypertension following buproprion overdose should be treated with benzodiazepines for seizure prophylaxis.

C. Monoamine Oxidase Inhibitor Overdose and Drug and Food Interactions

1. Treat behavioral hyperactivity with benzodiazepines. Intubation and neuromuscular paralysis (along with cooling measures) may be necessary in patients with hyperthermia.

2. Treat hypertension and tachycardia only if severe. Use easily titratable and reversible agents such as IV nitroprusside and esmolol.
3. Treat hypotension with direct-acting vasopressors such as epinephrine and norepinephrine; avoid dopamine.
4. MAOI overdose requires admission to the ICU for at least 24 hours, even in the absence of symptoms, because toxicity can be delayed.

D. Serotonin Syndrome

1. Generally responds to withdrawal of the causative agent(s) and supportive care.
2. Administer benzodiazepines to reduce motor activity and control hyperthermia. As with MAOIs, neuromuscular paralysis and intubation may become necessary.
3. Cyproheptadine, a selective 5-HT$_{2A}$ antagonist, may be beneficial. Administer an initial dose of 8 mg (by mouth or gastric tube). Repeat dose if symptoms do not improve after 2 hours or if symptoms recur. The maximum dose is 24 mg per day.
4. Symptoms usually resolve in 24 to 48 hours.

IV. COMPLICATIONS

A. Pulmonary aspiration, pneumonia, rhabdomyolysis, and sepsis are common in patients with coma and seizures.
B. Shock or anoxia can result in multiple-organ dysfunction.
C. Hypertensive crisis from MAOI interactions can result in intracranial hemorrhage.

Selected Readings

Boehnert M, Lovejoy FH Jr. Value of the QRS duration versus the serum drug level in predicting seizures and ventricular arrhythmias after an acute overdose of tricyclic antidepressants. *N Engl J Med* 1985;313:474–479.
This paper correlates the degree of QRS prolongation to the risk of subsequent seizures or cardiac dysrhythmia. This study provides the rationale for alkalinization of serum with a QRS duration of longer than 100 msec.

Linden CH, Rumack BH, Strehlke C. Monoamine oxidase inhibitor overdose. *Ann Emerg Med* 1984;13(12):1137–1144.
An overview of the pathophysiology of, presentation of, and treatment for MAOI toxicity.

Sternbach H. The serotonin syndrome. *Am J Psychiatry* 1991;148:705–713.
This is a landmark review of 38 cases of serotonin syndrome from which a set of diagnostic criteria was developed known as the Sternbach criteria.

Tokarski GF, Young MJ. Criteria for admitting patients with tricyclic antidepressant overdose. *J Emerg Med* 1998;6:121–124.
Provides a review of tricyclic antidepressant toxicity and the rationale for determining patient disposition.

ANTIHYPERTENSIVE AGENTS
Ivan E. Liang

8

I. BACKGROUND

A. The antihypertensive agents discussed in this chapter are generally less toxic than β-adrenergic and calcium channel blockers (see Chapters 11 and 12).

B. Manifestations of overdosage are the result of exaggerated pharmacological activity.

II. PATHOPHYSIOLOGY

A. Loop Diuretics

1. Loop diuretics (Table 8-1) decrease renal water reabsorption, increase renal blood flow, and enhance solute (e.g., sodium, chloride, potassium, hydrogen ion, calcium, magnesium, ammonium, bicarbonate, phosphate) excretion. Acutely, they increase venous capacitance by dilating large veins.

2. Auditory toxicity is enhanced when these agents are used with aminoglycosides and cisplatin.

3. Injectable formulations for parenteral use are available for furosemide and bumetanide.

B. Thiazide and Related Diuretics

1. Thiazides (Table 8-2) enhance renal excretion of sodium, chloride, and water.

2. Acutely, they lower the blood pressure by reducing plasma volume and cardiac output.

3. They should be used with caution in patients with renal disease.

4. Thiazide-induced hypokalemia and hypomagnesemia can predispose to cardiac glycoside toxicity.

5. Other side effects include hyperglycemia, hypercalcemia, and hyperuricemia.

6. Acute single ingestions rarely cause any toxic manifestations.

C. Potassium-sparing Diuretics

1. These drugs (Table 8-3) enhance the effects of other diuretics and counteract their kaluretic action.

2. Overdose may result in hyperkalemia, especially in patients with renal impairment.

3. Concurrent administration of angiotensin-converting enzyme inhibitors or potassium can also result in hyperkalemia.

TABLE 8-1 Dosing Guidelines for the Loop Diuretics in the Treatment of Hypertension

	Furosemide[a-c]	Bumetanide[a-c]	Torsemide[a-c]	Ethacrynic acid[a-c]
Starting dose	10–20 mg p.o. b.i.d.	0.5 mg p.o. q.d.	5 mg p.o. q.d.	25–50 mg p.o. q.d.
Usual maintenance dose	20–40 mg p.o. b.i.d.	1–2 mg p.o. q.d.	5–10 mg p.o. q.d.	25–50 mg p.o. b.i.d.
Maximum dose	160–240 mg p.o. b.i.d.	5 mg p.o. b.i.d.	10 mg q.d.	100 mg p.o. b.i.d.
Relative potency	1	~40	~4	0.6–0.8

Source: Irwin RS, Rippe JM. *Manual of Intensive Care Medicine*, 3rd ed. Philadelphia: Lippincott Williams & Wilkins, 2000:596.
[a]The hypotensive effect of antihypertensive agents may be enhanced during concomitant loop diuretic administration. The dosage of the antihypertensive agent should be reduced when a loop diuretic is added to an existing antihypertensive regimen.
[b]The loop diuretics are contraindicated in patients with anuria.
[c]Patients with renal disease and liver disease may require higher doses of the loop diuretics.
p.o., by mouth; b.i.d., twice daily; q.d., every day.

TABLE 8-2   **Available Preparations and the Oral Dosing Guidelines for the Thiazide and Related Diuretics for the Treatment of Hypertension**

Diuretic	Preparations	Starting dose	Maintenance dose	Maximal dose (mg)
Chlorothiazide	250, 500/mg tablets; 250 mg/5 mL oral suspension	250–500 mg/d	250–1000 mg/d	1,000
Hydrochlorothiazide	25, 50, 100 mg tablets; 50 mg/5 mL, 100 mg/mL oral solution	50–100 mg/d	25–100 mg/d	200
Bendroflumethiazide	5, 10 mg tablets	5–20 mg/d	2.5–15 mg/d	20
Cyclothiazide	2 mg tablets	2 mg/d	2–4 mg/d	6
Methyclothiazide	2.5, 5 mg tablets	2.5–5 mg/d	2.5–5 mg/d	5
Benzthiazide	50 mg tablets	25–50 mg b.i.d.	25–50 mg b.i.d.	200
Hydroflumethiazide	50 mg tablets	50 mg b.i.d.	50–100 mg/d	200
Trichlormethiazide	2, 4 tablets	2 mg/d	2–4 mg/d	4
Polythiazide	1, 2, 4 mg tablets	2 mg/d	1–4 mg/d	4
Quinethazone	50 mg tablets	50–100 mg/d	50–100 mg/d	200
Metolazone	2.5, 5, 10 mg extended tablets 0.5 mg prompt tablets	2.5–5 mg/d 0.5 mg/d	2.5–5 mg/d 0.5–1 mg/d	10 1
Chlorthalidone	25, 50, 100 mg tablets	25 mg/d	25–50 mg/d	100
Indapamide	2.5 mg tablets	2.5 mg/d	2.5–5 mg/d	5

Source: Irwin RS, Rippe JM. *Manual of Intensive Care Medicine*, 3rd ed Philadelphia: Lippincott Williams & Wilkins, 2000:597.

| TABLE 8-3 | Dosing Guidelines for the Potassium-Sparing Diuretics |

	Spironolactone[a,b]	Triamterene[a,b]	Amiloride[a,b]
Starting dose	25–100 mg p.o. q.d.	50–100 mg p.o. b.i.d.	5 mg p.o. q.d.
Usual maintenance dose	50–100 mg p.o. q.d.	50–100 mg p.o. q.d.–b.i.d.	5–10 mg p.o. q.d.
Maximal dose	200 mg p.o. q.d.	150 mg p.o. b.i.d.	20 mg p.o. q.d.

Source: Irwin RS, Rippe JM. *Manual of Intensive Care Medicine,* 3rd ed. Philadelphia: Lippincott Williams & Wilkins, 2000:598.
[a]Take with food.
[b]When used in conjunction with other diuretics, reducing the doses of these agents may be required.
p.o., orally; q.d., every day; b.i.d., twice daily.

D. Angiotensin-converting Enzyme (ACE) Inhibitors

1. ACE inhibitors (Table 8-4) also inhibit bradykinin metabolism and enhance prostaglandin synthesis, which contribute to unwanted side effects such as cough, urticaria, and angioedema.
2. These side effects may occur anytime during therapy. Angioedema can result in airway compromise.
3. Patients with sodium or volume depletion and those taking diuretics are at increased risk for hypotension and renal failure as well as for hyperkalemia.

E. Angiotensin II Receptor Antagonists (ARBs)

1. ARBs (Table 8-5) block angiotensin II–type 1 receptors, resulting in vasodilation, decreased aldosterone secretion, and enhanced sodium and water excretion.
2. The toxicity of ARBs is very similar to that of ACE inhibitors.
3. Although less common than with ACE inhibitors, angioedema has been reported after use of ARBs and is more likely in patients who experienced angioedema while taking ACE inhibitors.

F. Centrally Active Antiadrenergic Agents

1. These agents (Table 8-6) decrease central sympathetic outflow by stimulating presynaptic α_2-adrenergic receptors in the brain.
2. Most overdoses involve clonidine, perhaps because of its widespread use, low price, and use in the treatment of attention deficit hyperactivity disorder and opioid withdrawal.
   a. Toxicity is characterized by pupillary constriction, central nervous system (CNS) depression (lethargy, coma), bradycardia, and hypotension.
   b. Transient peripheral α_1-receptor stimulation with paradoxical sympathomimetic effects may occur early in the course of poisoning.
   c. Symptoms typically develop within 30 to 60 minutes of ingestion, peak as late as 6 to 12 hours, and resolve by 24 hours.

TABLE 8-4 Dosing Guidelines for the Angiotensin-Converting Enzyme (ACE) Inhibitors

Drug	Initial dose	Maintenance dose	Hypodynamic	Hyperdynamic
Benazepril	10 mg q.d.	20–80 mg q.d.	Reduce doses	10 mg q.d., titrate upward, divide b.i.d. if response diminished at end of dosing interval
Captopril	12.5–25 mg b.i.d.-t.i.d.	25–150 mg/d divided b.i.d. or t.i.d	Reduce doses	25 mg t.i.d., titrate upward to response
Enalapril	5 mg q.d.	10–40 mg/d divided q.d. or b.i.d.	Reduce doses	5 mg q.d., titrate upward, divide b.i.d. if response diminished at end of dosing interval
Enalaprilat	1.25 mg IV q6h	2.5 mg IV q6h	Begin 0.625 mg IV q6h; however, a 18q dosing interval may be required in some cases	1.25 mg IV q6h, titrate upward to response
Fosinopril	10 mg q.d.	20–80 mg q.d.	No change	10 mg q.d., titrate to response, divide b.i.d. if response diminished at end of dosing interval
Lisinopril	10 mg q.d.	20–40 mg q.d.	Reduce doses	10 mg q.d., titrate to response
Moexipril	7.5 mg q.d.	7.5–60 mg q.d. divided q.d. or b.i.d.	Reduce doses	7.5 mg q.d., titrate to response, divide b.i.d. if response diminished at end of dosing interval
Quinapril	10 mg q.d.	20–80 mg/d divided q.d. or b.i.d.	Reduce doses	10 mg q.d., titrate to response, divide b.i.d. if response is diminished at end of dosing interval
Ramipril	2.5 mg q.d.	2.5–20 mg/d divided q.d. or b.i.d.	Reduce doses	2.5 mg q.d., titrate to response, divide b.i.d. if response is diminished at end of dosing interval
Trandolapril	1–2 mg q.d.	2–8 mg/d divided q.d. or b.i.d.	Reduce doses	1–2 mg q.d., titrate to response divide b.i.d. if response is diminished at end of dosing interval

Source: Irwin RS, Rippe JM. Manual of Intensive Care Medicine, 3rd ed. Philadelphia: Lippincott Williams & Wilkins, 2000:599.
q.d., every day; b.i.d., twice daily; t.i.d., three times a day; IV, intravenous.

TABLE 8-5	Dosing Guidelines for Angiotensin II Antagonists			
Agent	Initial dose	Maintenance dose	Hypodynamic	Hyperdynamic
Losartan (CoZaar)	25–50 mg q.d.	25–100 mg/d divided q.d. or b.i.d.	Begin with 25 mg q.d., titrate to response	50 mg q.d., titrate to response, divided b.i.d. if response diminished at end of dosing interval
Valsartan (Diovan)	80 mg q.d.	80–320 mg q.d.	No change	80 mg q.d., titrate to response
Irbesartan (Avapro)	150 mg q.d.	150–300 mg q.d.	No change	150 mg q.d., titrate to response

Source: Irwin RS, Rippe JM. *Manual of Intensive Care Medicine,* 3rd ed. Philadelphia: Lippincott Williams & Wilkins, 2000:600.
q.d., every day; b.i.d., twice daily.

    d. Rebound effects (hypertension and sympathomimetic symptoms) often occur after abrupt discontinuation of chronic use.

    e. Immidazoline nasal decongestants (e.g., oxymetazoline, tetrahydrozoline) have similar structure and toxicity.

G. Nitroglycerin

    1. Nitroglycerin relaxes vascular smooth muscle by increasing cyclic guanosine monophosphate. The venous circulation is affected most.

    2. Vasodilatory effects can be greatly potentiated when combined with sildenafil and related agents used for erectile dysfunction (vardenafil and tadalafil).

    3. Toxic effects include headache, skin flushing, and hypotension (markedly orthostatic) with reflex tachycardia.

H. Nitroprusside

    1. Nitroprusside is a vasodilator that can cause hypotension and reflex tachycardia.

    2. It is metabolized to cyanide, which combines with thiosulfate to form thiocyanate. Thiocyanate is eliminated by the kidneys.

    3. Cyanide toxicity can occur when thiosulfate body stores are depleted. It is most likely to occur early in treatment, at elevated doses, and in patients with poor nutrition, chronic disease, recent surgery, or chronic diuretic use.

        a. Manifestations of cyanide poisoning include agitation, seizures, tachypnea, hypotension, dysrhythmias, and lactic acidemia.

        b. Hydroxycobalamin (25 mg/h intravenously [IV]) administered with nitroprusside can prevent this complication.

    4. Thiocyanate can accumulate in patients with renal insufficiency and prolonged treatment. Manifestations of thiocyanate toxicity include agitation, delusions, disorientation, tremors, seizures, and coma.

TABLE 8-6 Dosing Guidelines for the α_2 Receptor Agonists

	Oral clonidine[a,b]	Transdermal clonidine[a,b]	Oral methyldopa[a,b]	Injectable methyldopa[a,b]	Oral guanabenz[a,b]	Oral guanfacine[b]
Starting dose	0.1 mg b.i.d.	One No. 1 patch weekly	250 mg b.i.d.	250 mg–1 g IV q6h	4 mg b.i.d.	1 mg at bedtime
Usual maintenance dose	0.3 mg b.i.d.	One No. 1–No. 3 patch weekly	500 mg–2 g/d in 2–4 doses	250 mg–1 g IV q6h	16 mg b.i.d.	1–3 mg q.d.
Maximal dose	2.4 mg/day	Two No. 3 patches weekly	2 g/d	250 mg–1 g IV q6h	32 mg b.i.d.	3 mg q.d.

Source: Irwin RS, Rippe JM. *Manual of Intensive Care Medicine*, 3rd ed. Philadelphia: Lippincott Williams & Wilkins, 2000:601

[a]Dosage adjustment necessary in patients with severe renal dysfunction.
[b]Dosage adjustment may be necessary in patients with severe hepatic failure.
b.i.d., twice daily; IV, intravenous.

TABLE 8-7	Dosing Guidelines for the α_1-Adrenergic Blockers		

	Prazosin[a-c]	Terazosin[c]	Doxazosin[c]
Starting dose	1 mg b.i.d.–t.i.d.	1 mg/d	1 mg/d
Usual maintenance dose	2–20 mg/d (divided doses)	1–20 mg/d	1–16 mg/d
Maximal dose	20–40 mg/d (divided doses)	20 mg/d	16 mg/d

Source: Irwin RS, Rippe JM. *Manual of Intensive Care Medicine,* 3rd ed. Philadelphia: Lippincott Williams & Wilkins, 2000:602.
[a]Take the first dose at bedtime.
[b]Patients with renal failure may require smaller doses.
[c]Dosage adjustments may be necessary in patients with severe liver failure.
b.i.d., orally; t.i.d., three times daily.

5. Elevated whole blood cyanide or serum thiocyanate concentrations confirm these diagnoses.

I. α_1-Adrenergic Blockers
1. These drugs (Table 8-7) produce arterial and venous dilation, resulting in hypotension and reflex tachycardia after overdose.
2. Side effects include lassitude, vivid dreams, and depression.
3. A "first dose" phenomenon (transient dizziness, palpitations, and syncope) can occur within 1 to 3 hours after the first dose.

J. Vasodilators
1. These agents (Table 8-8) cause arteriolar dilation with reflex tachycardia and activation of the renin–angiotensin system.
2. If used alone, these agents can precipitate myocardial ischemia in patients with underlying coronary artery disease.
3. Minoxidil is also used as a topical treatment for hair loss.

TABLE 8-8	Dosing Guidelines for Hydralazine and Minoxidil	

	Hydralazine[a-c]	Minoxidil[c]
Starting dose	10 mg q.i.d. p.o.	5 mg q.d. p.o.
Usual maintenance dose	10–50 mg q.i.d. p.o.	10–40 mg/d p.o.
Maximal dose	300 mg/d p.o.	100 mg/d p.o.

Source: Irwin RS, Rippe JM. *Manual of Intensive Care Medicine,* 3rd ed. Philadelphia: Lippincott Williams & Wilkins, 2000:602.
[a]Take with meals (food enhances bioavailability).
[b]Dosage adjustments necessary in patients with moderate to severe renal dysfunction.
[c]Dosage adjustments may be necessary in patients with severe hepatic failure.
q.i.d., four times daily; p.o., orally.

III. DIAGNOSIS

A. Most acute ingestions result in limited toxicity, except for clonidine and except in those with underlying cardiovascular disease.

B. Overdose effects are generally nonspecific, and the diagnosis is made from the exposure history.

C. Orthostatic hypotension is common and can occur with therapeutic doses.

D. Severe poisoning can cause supine hypotension; reflex tachycardia is common, except with centrally acting α_2-blockers.

E. Agent-specific effects include:

    1. Hypokalemia and hypomagnesemia from loop and thiazide diuretics.

    2. Hyperkalemia from potassium-sparing diuretics.

    3. Angioedema from ACE inhibitors (can be confused with acute hypersensitivity reactions).

    4. Opioid effects from clonidine (see Chapter 29).

    5. Cyanide and thiocyanate toxicity from nitroprusside.

F. Evaluation of patients with hypotension should include an electrocardiogram (ECG); cardiac monitoring; and serum electrolytes, blood urea nitrogen (BUN), creatinine, magnesium, and other laboratory tests as clinically indicated.

IV. TREATMENT

A. Treatment is supportive and directed toward treating hypotension and reversing electrolyte abnormalities after addressing the airway.

B. Hypotension may be initially treated with fluid boluses followed by IV pressors (dopamine, 5 to 15 mcg/kg/min, or norepinephrine, 0.1 mcg/kg/min).

C. Activated charcoal should be considered for recent oral overdoses (see Chapter 1).

D. Angioedema can be treated with ice, antihistamines, corticosteroids, and epinephrine (for severe cases), but the response is slow and variable.

E. Clonidine toxicity inconsistently responds to high-dose naloxone (4 to 10 mg IV in adults).

F. Treatment of cyanide toxicity from nitroprusside includes discontinuation of the drug and administration of sodium thiosulfate (see Chapter 34). Hemodialysis can effectively remove thiocyanate.

V. COMPLICATIONS

A. Profound or prolonged hypotension can cause hypoperfusion of end organs such as the heart, central nervous system, and kidneys, resulting in myocardial ischemia and infarction, stroke, and renal failure.

B. Severe electrolyte abnormalities result in cardiac arrhythmias.

Selected Readings

Curry SC, Arnold-Capell P. Toxic effects of drugs used in the ICU. Nitroprusside, nitroglycerin, and angiotensin-converting enzyme inhibitors. *Crit Care Clin* 1991; 7(3):555–581.

A discussion of cyanide toxicity associated with nitroprusside use.

Howes LG, Tran D. Can angiotensin receptor antagonists be used safely in patients with previous ACE inhibitor–induced angioedema? *Drug Saf* 2002;25(2):73–76.
Review of both ACE inhibitor– and angiotensin receptor antagonist–induced angioedema.

Seger DL. Clonidine toxicity revisited. *J Toxicol Clin Toxicol* 2002;40(2):145–155.
A review of clonidine poisoning and treatment.

ANTIMICROBIAL AGENTS
D. Eric Brush

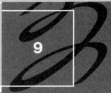

9

I. BACKGROUND

A. Antimicrobials are chemically diverse medications used to treat infections of bacteria, viruses, fungi, or protozoa and occasionally for noninfectious conditions.

B. They are most notable for producing various adverse effects and drug–drug interactions in therapeutic dosing, rather than causing toxicity in overdose.

C. Gastrointestinal (GI) irritation is the most common manifestation of oral overdose.

D. Agent-specific adverse effects with therapeutic dosing and overdose are wide ranging and include cardiac dysrhythmias, hematologic abnormalities, and seizures.

II. PATHOPHYSIOLOGY

A. Antibacterial Agents

1. Penicillins, cephalosporins, and other β-lactams

 a. Inhibit bacterial cell wall synthesis.

 b. In high intravenous (IV) doses (>50 million U/day) penicillin G can cause seizures via γ-aminobutyric acid (GABA) antagonism.

 c. Imipenem may also cause seizures through a similar mechanism.

 d. Other adverse effects include immune-mediated toxicity, such as interstitial nephritis, bone marrow suppression, vasculitis, rash, and Stevens–Johnson syndrome.

 e. Cephalosporins with the nMTT side chain (cefazolin, cefotetan, moxalactam, cefmetazole, cefamandole, and cefoperazone) can interact with ethanol to produce a disulfuramlike reaction (nausea, vomiting, flushing, headache, and, rarely, hypotension and shock).

2. Tetracycline

 a. Inhibits 30S and 50S bacterial ribosomes and thus protein synthesis.

 b. Adverse effects include photosensitivity dermatitis, pseudotumor cerebri, and neuromuscular blockade in patients with myasthenia gravis.

 c. Use after the first 12 weeks of gestation or in the first 8 years of life leads to permanent staining of secondary teeth.

3. Macrolides (erythromycin, clarithromycin, and azithromycin)

 a. Inhibit bacterial 50S ribosomes and protein synthesis.

    b. An adverse effect from the estolate formulation of erythromycin is cholestatic jaundice.

    c. Erythromycin and clarithromycin inhibit cytochrome P-450 3A4 and 1A2 and can increase warfarin, theophylline, carbamazepine, and cyclosporine concentrations. They also induce p-glycoprotein–facilitated drug transport and can increase digoxin levels.

    d. Intravenous erythromycin may lead to QTc prolongation and torsades de pointes (TdP).

4. Lincosamides (lincomycin and clindamycin)

    a. Act by inhibiting bacterial protein synthesis similar to macrolides.

    b. Adverse effects include GI irritation and pseudomembranous colitis.

5. Sulfonamides

    a. Inhibit bacterial folate synthesis, thereby halting nucleic acid production.

    b. Have a high incidence of allergic reactions.

    c. Adverse effects include hemolysis and/or methemoglobinemia (see Chapter 34), nephrotoxicity from crystal formation, and bone marrow suppression.

6. Trimethoprim

    a. Inhibits bacterial folate synthesis and works synergistically with sulfonamides.

    b. Adverse effects include bone marrow suppression.

7. Chloramphenicol

    a. Inhibits bacterial 50S ribosomes and protein synthesis.

    b. Adverse effects include fatal bone marrow suppression.

    c. Decreased hepatic metabolism in neonates and infants can result in the gray baby syndrome, which is characterized by ashen color, metabolic acidosis, vomiting, tachypnea, lethargy, and cardiovascular collapse.

    d. Cardiovascular collapse may occur up to 12 hours after overdose.

8. Vancomycin

    a. Inhibits bacterial glycopeptidase polymerase, preventing cell wall synthesis.

    b. Adverse effects include ototoxicity and nephrotoxicity, particularly with excessive dosing.

    c. Rapid IV infusion can cause an anaphylactoid reaction with generalized flushing called the "red man syndrome." Severe hypotension and cardiac arrest have also been reported.

9. Linezolid

    a. Inhibits bacterial 50S ribosomes and protein synthesis.

    b. Inhibits monoamine oxidase and may cause hypertensive crisis with ingestion of tyramine-containing foods or serotonin syndrome if patient is on serotonergic medications (see Chapter 7).

    c. Adverse effects include bone marrow suppression.

10. Metronidazole

    a. May form toxic metabolites within bacteria and protozoa.

    b. Adverse effects include GI distress and disulfuramlike reactions with ethanol. Reversible peripheral neuropathy may also occur.

11. Fluoroquinolones
  a. Inhibit bacterial DNA topoisomerase and gyrase.
  b. Inhibit K^+ channels in the myocardium and can cause QTc prolongation.
  c. Fatal hepatotoxicity has occurred with trovafloxacin.
  d. Psychosis and seizures can occur with therapeutic doses as well as with overdose.
  e. Chondrotoxicity has caused spontaneous Achilles tendon rupture. Use should be avoided in pregnancy and childhood because of concerns for developing cartilage.
12. Aminoglycosides
  a. Inhibit bacterial 30S ribosomal subunit and protein synthesis.
  b. Adverse effects include permanent ototoxicity.
  c. Nephrotoxicity is also common and is related to the length of time that serum concentrations remain elevated. Once daily dosing decreases this effect.
  d. Neuromuscular weakness may result from inhibition of acetylcholine release at the neuromuscular junction as well as acetylcholine receptor antagonism. This effect can be significant in patients with myasthenia gravis and those treated with paralytic agents and corticosteroids.
13. Isoniazid (INH)
  a. Inhibits enzymes required for the synthesis of mycobacterial cell walls (mycolic acids).
  b. Toxicity in overdose is characterized by refractory seizures, acidosis, and persistent coma (see Chapter 23).
14. Dapsone
  a. Likely inhibits folic acid synthesis.
  b. Adverse effects include GI upset, fever, rash, and methemoglobinemia (see Chapter 34).

B. Antiviral Agents
  1. Acyclovir
    a. Inhibits viral nucleic acid synthesis.
    b. Parenteral administration may cause delirium, tremor, seizures, hypotension, and nephrotoxicity (crystal deposition).
  2. Amantadine
    a. Prevents viral penetration into host cells.
    b. Enhances dopaminergic neurotransmission and has anticholinergic activity.
    c. Overdose may lead to anticholinergic toxicity, QTc and QRS prolongation, and delirium.
  3. Foscarnet
    a. Inhibits herpes virus DNA polymerase.
    b. GI upset limits oral administration.
    c. IV administration may cause hypocalcemia, hypophosphatemia, hypomagnesemia, and hypokalemia.
    d. Seizures and renal failure can also occur.
  4. Nucleoside analogs
    a. Inhibit reverse transcription of viral nucleic acids.

   b. Adverse effects include lactic acidosis.
   c. Zidovudine (AZT) can cause anemia and granulocytopenia.
   d. Didanosine can cause pancreatitis and peripheral neuropathy.
  5. Protease inhibitors
   a. Prevent the cleavage of viral proteins.
   b. Common adverse effects include GI upset and diarrhea.
   c. Agent-specific effects include nephrolithiasis (indinavir), neutropenia (nelfinavir), and peripheral neuropathy (saquinavir).

C. Antifungal Agents
  1. Amphotericin B
   a. Binds to ergosterol, a component of fungal cell membranes, leading to pore formation which disrupts the membrane.
   b. Common adverse effects include fever, rigors, vomiting, headache, and nephrotoxicity.
   c. Hypotension, hypokalemia, shock, and ventricular fibrillation have also been reported.
  2. Flucytosine
   a. Metabolized to fluorouracil (5-FU), which disrupts fungal nucleic acid synthesis via thymidylate synthase.
   b. Adverse effects include bone marrow suppression, peripheral neuropathies, and seizures.
  3. Griseofulvin
   a. Inhibits fungal microtubule formation.
   b. Adverse effects include hypersensitivity reactions, headaches, and confusion.
  4. Azoles (fluconazole, itraconazole, ketoconazole)
   a. Inhibit the formation of ergosterol, which is needed for fungal cell membrane synthesis.
   b. Inhibit cytochrome CYP3A4, leading to increased plasma levels of antiarrhythmics, coumadin, phenytoin, and other drugs.
   c. Other adverse effects include GI toxicity and hepatotoxicity.

D. Antiprotozoal Agents
  1. Chloroquine
   a. Selectively disrupts protozoal cell membranes.
   b. Blocks Na^+ and K^+ channels in the central nervous system (CNS) and myocardium (see Chapter 4).
   c. Overdose can cause seizures, refractory hypotension, hypokalemia, TdP, and ventricular fibrillation (VF).
  2. Quinine
   a. Prevents DNA replication by preventing the unbinding of DNA for transcription.
   b. Can cause cinchonism, which is characterized by headache, vertigo, hearing loss, blurred vision, and tinnitus (see Chapter 4).
   c. Overdose may cause quinidine-like toxicity due to Na^+ and K^+ channel blockade (see Chapter 4).
   d. Adverse effects include methemoglobinemia and/or hemolysis.
   e. Seizures and ventricular dysrhythmias including ventricular tachycardia (VT), VF, and TdP may occur.

    f. Mefloquine is structurally and pharmacologically similar to quinine but is less toxic.
  3. Primaquine
    a. Metabolized to cellular oxidants within malaria parasites.
    b. Adverse effects include methemoglobinemia and/or hemolysis.
  4. Pyrimethamine
    a. Inhibits protozoal dihydrofolate reductase.
    b. Can cause folate deficiency and megaloblastic anemia.
    c. Seizures, blindness, deafness, and mental retardation have occurred in children following overdose.
    d. Proguanil has a similar mechanism and is synergistic in its effect on folate metabolism.
  5. Pentamidine
    a. Interferes with nucleic acid synthesis in trypanosomes.
    b. Hypotension, QTc prolongation, TdP, and VF have occurred with IV administration. Iatrogenic overdose has caused hypotension and cardiac arrest.
    c. Adverse effects include nephrotoxicity and pancreatic β cell dysfunction.

III. DIAGNOSIS

  A. The diagnosis of adverse drug-related events relies primarily on the history because most antimicrobial agents do not have easily recognized patterns of toxicity.
  B. Evaluation of patients with adverse therapeutic effects or overdose should include a complete blood count (CBC), electrolytes, blood urea nitrogen (BUN), creatinine, and glucose.
    1. Patients exposed to agents with cardiovascular or neurological toxicity should have an electrocardiogram (ECG; with attention to conduction intervals) and serum calcium, magnesium, and phosphate levels tested.
    2. Liver function tests should be obtained with hepatotoxic drug exposure.
    3. Patients exposed to agents that have drug–drug interactions and who are taking medications such as warfarin, digoxin, and phenytoin should have coagulation studies done or specific drug concentrations measured.
    4. Patients treated with prolonged courses of aminoglycosides and vancomycin should have their serum drug concentrations monitored.

IV. TREATMENT

  A. The majority of adverse events related to therapeutic use or overdose with antimicrobials are treated with removal of the drug and supportive care.
  B. Patients with cardiovascular or neurological toxicity should have IV access and cardiac monitoring established.
    1. Advanced life support measures should be instituted as necessary.
    2. Seizures can be managed with benzodiazepines and/or barbiturates.
  C. Activated charcoal should be administered for recent oral overdose (see Chapter 1).

D. Specific treatments include:
1. Methylene blue for methemoglobinemia resulting from sulfonamide, dapsone, and antiprotozoal agents (see Chapter 34).
2. Cardiac monitoring for at least 12 hours for large overdoses of chloramphenicol. Consider hemodialysis for massive overdose, decreased ability to eliminate the drug (hepatic or renal failure), or severe cardiac compromise.
3. Stopping the infusion and administering diphenhydramine for vancomycin-associated red man syndrome. The infusion can be resumed at a slower rate after symptoms resolve.
4. Treatment of the serotonin syndrome or hypertensive crisis caused by linezolid as for other causes (see Chapter 7).
5. Intravenous pyridoxine for INH overdose (see Chapter 23).
6. Sodium bicarbonate for cardiac conduction delays and arrhythmias (see Chapter 4), and physostigmine for anticholinergic poisoning from amantadine (see Chapter 5).
7. Exchange transfusion for amphotericin B toxicity resulting from large iatrogenic overdose in infants and neonates.
8. High-dose diazepam (2 mg/kg IV over 30 min followed by 1 to 2 mg/kg/day for up to 4 days) for CNS and cardiac toxicity from chloroquine overdose.
   a. Sodium bicarbonate for cardiac conduction delays and arrhythmias (see Chapter 4).
   b. Epinephrine drip for hypotension refractory to IV fluids.
   c. Expectant monitoring of hypokalemia, which results from intracellular shifts and not total body deficit.
9. Sodium bicarbonate, lidocaine, magnesium, and cardiac pacing for conduction delays and arrhythmias caused by quinine (see Chapter 4).
10. Folate supplementation for prevention and treatment of pyrimethamine and proguanil hematologic toxicity.

Selected Readings

Riou B, Barriot P, Rimailho A, et al. Treatment of severe chloroquine poisoning. *N Engl J Med* 1988;318:1–6.
This is a prospective human trial using high-dose diazepam and epinephrine in the treatment of severe chloroquine poisoning. A significant decrease in mortality was noted.

Stahlmann R, Lode H. Toxicity of quinolones. *Drugs* 1999;58(suppl 2):37–42.
A review of the wide variety of available quinolones and their unique associated toxicities.

Wallace KL. Antibiotic-induced convulsions. *Med Toxicol* 1997;13:741–762.
This article provides an overview of the many antibiotics that may produce seizures.

ANTIPSYCHOTIC AGENTS

Steven B. Bird

10

I. BACKGROUND

A. Antipsychotic agents, also known as neuroleptics and major tranquilizers, include phenothiazines as well as a variety of other agents (Table 10-1).

B. They are primarily used in the therapy of schizophrenia, the manic phase of bipolar disorders, and agitated behavior.

C. They are also used as anesthesia adjuncts and to treat nausea, vomiting, headaches, and hiccups.

II. PATHOPHYSIOLOGY

A. Neuroleptics primarily act by binding to and blocking type 2 dopamine receptors (D_2) in the central nervous system (CNS).

B. They also have variable affinity for α-adrenergic, histamine, muscarinic, serotonergic, and other dopaminergic receptors.

C. Toxic effects include CNS and cardiovascular depression as well as anticholinergic, extrapyramidal, and neuroleptic malignant syndromes.

III. DIAGNOSIS

A. Clinical Effects Following Overdose

1. CNS and cardiovascular depression are usually evident within 1 to 2 hours of overdose, and maximal severity is apparent within 6 hours of ingestion.

2. Cardiovascular effects include hypotension, cardiac conduction disturbances, bradyarrhythmias, and ventricular tachyarrhythmias, including torsades de pointes.

3. Conduction disturbances include all degrees of atrioventricular (AV) block, bundle-branch block, and fascicular block and nonspecific intraventricular conduction delay.

4. Electrocardiographic changes (e.g., prolonged PR and QT intervals, ST-segment depression, T-wave abnormalities, U waves) and arrhythmias may be seen within several hours of overdose. Thioridazine, mesoridazine, and pimozide are responsible for the most fatal poisonings because of their greater cardiotoxicity.

TABLE 10-1 Neuroleptic Agents

Structural class	Generic name (trade name)	Affinity of neuroleptic agent for dopamine (D_2) receptor (potency)[a]	Daily dose range (mg)
Typical agents			
Butyrophenone	Droperidol (Inapsine)	3+	1.25–30.0
	Haloperidol (Haldol)	2+	1–30
Dihydroindolone	Molindone (Moban)	1+	15–225
Diphenylbutylpiperidine	Pimozide (Orap)	2+	1–20
Phenothiazine			
Aliphatic	Chlorpromazine (Thorazine)	2+	25–2,000
	Promazine (Sparine)[b]	–	50–1,000
	Promethazine (Phenergan)	2+	25–150
	Triflupromazine (Vesprin)	–	5–90
Piperazine	Fluphenazine (Prolixin)	3+	0.5–30.0
	Perphenazine (Trilafon)	3+	4–64
	Prochlorperazine (Compazine)	2+	10–150
	Trifluoperazine (Stelazine)	3+	2–40
Piperidine	Mesoridazine (Serentil)	2+	30–400
	Thioridazine (Mellaril, Millazine)	2+	20–800
Thioxanthene	Chlorprothixene (Taractan)	2+	30–600
	Flupenthixol[c]	3+	–
	Thiothixene (Navane)	3+	6–60
	Zuclopenthixol (Clopixol)[c]	3+	20–150
Atypical agents			
Benzamides	Amisulpiride[c]	2+	100–1,200
	Raclopride[c]	3+	5–8
	Remoxipride[c]	1+	150–600

TABLE 10-1 Neuroleptic Agents (*Continued*)

Structural class	Generic name (trade name)	Affinity of neuroleptic agent for dopamine (D$_2$) receptor (potency)[a]	Daily dose range (mg)
	Sulpride[c]	2+	100–1,600
	Trimethobenzamide (Tigan)[b]	–	100–600
Benzisothiazole	Ziprasidone (Geodon)	3+	40–160
Benzisoxazole	Risperidone (Risperdal)	3+	2–16
Dibenzodiazepine	Clozapine (Clozaril, Leponex)	1+	150–900
Dibenzoxazepine	Loxapine (Loxitane)	1+	20–250
Dibenzothiazepine	Quetiapine (Seroquel)	1+	300–600
Imidazolidinone	Sertindole (Serlect)[c]	3+	12–24
Thienobenzodiazepine	Olanzapine (Zyprexa)	2+	5–20

Source: Irwin RS, Rippe JM. *Irwin and Rippe's Intensive Care Medicine,* 5th ed. Philadelphia: Lippincott Williams & Wilkins, 2003:1531.
0, minimal to none; 1+, low; 2+, moderate; 3+, high to very high.
[a]A higher numerical value indicates greater binding affinity (greater antagonism) at D$_2$ receptor. Binding affinity (potency) at D$_2$ receptor correlates with daily dose range.
[b]Antiemetic only.
[c]Not available for clinical use in the United States.

5. Anticholinergic effects (see Chapter 5) are more common with atypical antipsychotic agents, which generally have increased antimuscarinic activity.

    a. Agitated delirium may appear as early as 30 minutes or as late as 24 hours after ingestion.

    b. Delirium, tachycardia, mydriasis, urinary retention, absence of bowel sounds, hyperthermia, and dry skin may be variably present.

6. Seizures, agitated delirium, loss of sweating ability, and hypothalamic dysfunction can cause hyperthermia.

7. Neuroleptic malignant syndrome (see later) rarely occurs following acute overdose. However, hypertension, hyperthermia, and hypertonia have been described.

8. Early deaths are caused by arrhythmias, shock, aspiration, and respiratory failure.

B. Adverse Effects of Therapeutic Doses

1. Extrapyramidal syndromes

    a. Result from the interference with dopaminergic function in the basal ganglia.

    b. Common with low-milligram, high-potency agents.

    c. Can occur early (hours to days), at an intermediate stage (days to months), or late (more than 3 months) in the course of therapy.

    d. Early extrapyramidal syndromes include acute dystonic reactions, intermediate syndromes include akathisia and parkinsonism, and late disorders include tardive dyskinesia and perioral tremor.

        (1) Acute dystonic reactions

            i. Characterized by abrupt onset, an intermittent and repetitive nature, normal physical examination except for muscular findings, a history of recent drug use, and rapid response to anticholinergic drug therapy.

            ii. Muscle contractions may be focal at the onset and then spread to contiguous muscles.

            iii. Patients remain alert and oriented. Muscles of the eye, face, tongue, neck, and torso can be involved.

            iv. Although these reactions are rarely life-threatening, those involving the tongue, jaw, and neck can result in upper airway compromise, impaired respiratory mechanics, and death.

        (2) Akathisia

            i. Can occur early after intravenous (IV) administration.

            ii. Manifestations include feelings of restlessness, tenseness, and difficulty in sitting still.

            iii. Examination may reveal agitation and motor hyperactivity with semipurposeful limb movements, especially of the legs and feet.

        (3) Drug-induced parkinsonism

            i. Indistinguishable from other causes of this syndrome except for the history of drug exposure.

            ii. Characterized by increased motor tone, decreased motor activity, tremors, and postural instability.

      iii. Tremors typically occur in the forearm and hand, are present at rest, worsen with agitation or excitement, and disappear with sleep.

      iv. Shuffling gait, cogwheel rigidity, limited upward gaze, and positive glabellar, snout, and sucking reflexes may be present.

2. Neuroleptic malignant syndrome (NMS)

  a. Idiosyncratic reaction that can be precipitated by intercurrent illness, surgery, dehydration, heat stress, and acute agitation.

  b. Onset is typically insidious and resolution occurs slowly, sometimes taking up to 2 weeks.

  c. Characterized by fever (higher than 38°C or 100.4°F), altered mental status (confusion, delirium, mutism, coma), autonomic dysfunction, increased motor activity, and laboratory abnormalities.

    (1) Autonomic disturbances include hypertension, tachycardia, tachypnea (or dyspnea, hypoxemia, or respiratory failure), diaphoresis (often profuse), and incontinence. Increased salivation, drooling, and hypotension may be seen.

    (2) Motor findings include "lead pipe" rigidity, akinesia, dystonia, dyskinesia, tremor, choreoid movements, opisthotonus, dysarthria, dysphagia, dysphonia, and trismus.

    (3) Laboratory abnormalities include leukocytosis, increased creatine phosphokinase (CPK), decreased serum iron, hypernatremia, hypokalemia, and syndrome of inappropriate secretion of antidiuretic hormone (SIADH).

C. Differential Diagnosis

1. Poisoning by alcohols, antiarrhythmics, anticholinergics, anticonvulsants, antihistamines, opioids, and sedative-hypnotic agents can cause CNS and cardiovascular effects similar to those resulting from overdose.

2. Acute dystonic reaction can be confused with seizures, cerebrovascular accidents, encephalitis, tetanus, hypocalcemia, and strychnine poisoning.

3. Manifestations of NMS are similar to those of the serotonin syndrome (Chapter 7).

IV. TREATMENT

A. Overdose

1. Patients with protracted hypotension, CNS depression or agitation, seizures, or arrhythmias should be admitted to an intensive care setting.

2. Hypotension should be treated with IV fluids initially and then with direct-acting vasopressors (e.g., norepinephrine, phenylephrine).

3. Sinus and supraventricular tachycardias rarely require treatment.

4. Ventricular tachycardia should be treated with lidocaine or electrical cardioversion, depending on hemodynamic stability.

5. Sodium bicarbonate (1 to 2 mEq/kg) infusion is recommended for patients with QRS intervals greater than 120 msec (see Chapter 4). Types Ia, Ic, and II antiarrhythmics should be avoided.

6. Torsades de pointes (polymorphic ventricular tachycardia) should be treated with intravenous magnesium or isoproterenol or overdrive pacing (see Chapter 4).

7. Symptomatic bradyarrhythmias should be treated with atropine, epinephrine, dopamine, and isoproterenol.

8. Seizures can be treated with benzodiazepines or short-acting barbiturates. The effectiveness of phenytoin for phenothiazine-induced seizures has not been established and this agent is not recommended for seizure management.

9. Activated charcoal should be considered for gastrointestinal decontamination in patients with recent acute overdose (see Chapter 1).

10. Most patients with neuroleptic poisoning recover completely within several hours to days, depending on the severity of toxicity.

B. Extrapyramidal Syndromes

1. Acute dystonic reactions are treated with anticholinergic agents.

    a. Administer benztropine mesylate (Cogentin, 1 to 2 mg) or diphenhydramine (Benadryl, 50 to 100 mg) parenterally or orally.

    b. After resolution of symptoms, oral therapy should be continued for another 48 to 72 hours to prevent relapse.

    c. Benzodiazepines can be used as adjunctive therapy if the anticholinergic agents are not effective.

2. Akathisia may be treated with anticholinergic agents (see earlier) and sedation with benzodiazepines if severe.

3. Neuroleptic-induced parkinsonism can be treated with benztropine, biperiden, diphenhydramine, or trihexyphenidyl. Long-term treatment with these agents is needed for patients who require continued neuroleptic therapy. Amantadine (100 to 400 mg/day orally) is also effective and has fewer side effects.

C. Anticholinergic Toxidrome

1. Physostigmine is superior to benzodiazepines in the reversal of delirium and causes fewer adverse effects (see Chapter 5).

2. Physostigmine should not be given if the QRS is greater than 100 msec on the electrocardiogram.

D. Neuroleptic Malignant Syndrome

1. The management of NMS consists of good supportive care aimed primarily at decreasing muscle hyperactivity, eliminating hyperthermia, and stopping the offending medication.

2. Early intubation should be considered, along with liberal use of benzodiazepines and a nondepolarizing neuromuscular blocking agent.

3. No well-controlled trials of antidotal therapy have been conducted.

    a. Bromocriptine (2.5 to 5 mg by mouth three times daily), a dopamine agonist, may be useful.

    b. Anecdotal reports of clinical response to dantrolene and amantadine exist. However, these agents should not be considered first-line therapy.

V. COMPLICATIONS

A. Complications of acute poisoning include cerebral and pulmonary edema, disseminated intravascular coagulation, renal failure, and infection.

B. Complications of NMS include aspiration pneumonia, coagulopathy, rhabdomyolysis, renal failure, myocardial infarction, heart failure, dysrhythmias, and venous thromboembolism.

Selected Readings

American College of Neuropharmacology—Food and Drug Administration Task Force. Neurologic syndromes associated with antipsychotic drug use. *N Engl J Med* 1973; 289:20–23.
This is a discussion of the movement disorders associated with the use of neuroleptic agents.

Arita M, Surawicz B. Electrophysiologic effects of phenothiazines on canine cardiac fibers. *J Pharmacol Exp Ther* 1973;184:619–630.
This study demonstrated increased sodium concentration to reverse thioridazine-induced repolarization abnormalities but not the depolarization effects.

Burns MJ. The pharmacology and toxicology of atypical antipsychotic agents. *J Toxicol Clin Toxicol* 2001;39:1–14.
An excellent review of the newer, atypical antipsychotic drugs.

Burns MJ, Linden CH, Graudins A. A comparison of physostigmine and benzodiazepines for the treatment of anticholinergic poisoning. *Ann Emerg Med* 2000;35: 374–381.
A retrospective comparison of anticholinergic poisoning demonstrating the superiority of physostigmine over benzodiazepines.

Gupta J, Lovejoy FH. Acute phenothiazine toxicity in childhood: a five-year survey. *Pediatrics* 1967;39:771–774.
This report discussed the manifestations of phenothiazine toxicity in children.

Huston JR, Bell GE. The effect of thioridazine and chlorpromazine on the electrocardiogram. *JAMA* 1966;198:134–138.
This article reported the electrocardiographic effects of neuroleptics to be similar to those of the type Ia antidysrhythmic agents.

Nierenberg D, Disch M, Manheimer E, et al. Facilitating prompt diagnosis and treatment of the neuroleptic malignant syndrome. *Clin Pharmacol Ther* 1991;50: 580–586.
This review discussed the factors contributing to neuroleptic malignant syndrome.

Rosebush PI, Stewart T, Mazurek MF. The treatment of neuroleptic malignant syndrome: are dantrolene and bromocriptine useful adjuncts to supportive care? *Br J Psychiatry* 1991;159:709–712.
This small study demonstrated supportive therapy to be more beneficial than dantrolene or bromocriptine in the treatment of neuroleptic malignant syndrome.

Rupniak NM, Jenner P, Marsden CD. Acute dystonia induced by neuroleptic drugs. *Psychopharmacology* 1986;88:403–419.
This review discussed the cause and occurrence of dystonia during drug therapy.

Shalev A, Hermesh H, Munitz H. Mortality from neuroleptic malignant syndrome. *J Clin Psychiatry* 1989;50:18–25.
This review discussed the factors attributed to the decrease in mortality from neuroleptic malignant syndrome.

Sternbach H. The serotonin syndrome. *Am J Psychiatry* 1991;148:705–713.
The sentinel review of the serotonin syndrome.

Vassallo SU, Delaney KA. Pharmacologic effects on thermoregulation: mechanisms of drug-related heatstroke. *J Toxicol Clin Toxicol* 1989;27:199–224.
This review discussed the supportive management of neuroleptic malignant syndrome.

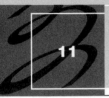

β-BLOCKER POISONING
Steven B. Bird

I. BACKGROUND

A. β-Blockers include a variety of agents that block β-adrenergic receptors of the peripheral nervous system (Table 11-1).

B. The incidence and severity of β-blocker poisoning have increased dramatically in recent years.

II. PATHOPHYSIOLOGY

A. β-Blockers competitively inhibit the binding of epinephrine and norepinephrine to G-protein–coupled β-adrenergic receptors in the heart, kidneys, and eyes (β_1 receptors); blood vessels, bronchioles, liver, and pancreas (β_2 receptors); and other organs.

B. Binding to the β receptors activates phosphodiesterase and increases cyclic adenosine monophosphate (cAMP).

C. Cardioselective β-blockers preferentially block β_1 receptors, some have β agonist activity, and some have sodium channel blocking, antiarrhythmic, or membrane-stabilizing effects (see Chapter 4 and Table 11-1).

D. β-Blockers are rapidly absorbed after oral ingestion.

    1. Toxicity can develop as early as 20 minutes after an overdose of an immediate-release preparation, with peak effects at 1 to 2 hours.

    2. Sustained-release formulations may be slowly absorbed, especially after overdose.

    3. Delayed toxicity can occur with sustained-release preparations and can last for several days.

E. The dose required to produce toxicity is highly variable and depends on the sympathetic tone and metabolic capacity of the patient and the pharmacologic and pharmacokinetic properties of the specific β-blocker.

F. The half-life can be greatly prolonged in patients with depressed cardiac output, resulting in decreased hepatic and renal perfusion. Intrinsic heart, kidney, and liver disease as well as the concomitant use of drugs with similar activity increases the risk of toxicity.

G. Pharmacokinetic data on individual agents are presented in Table 11-1.

III. DIAGNOSIS

A. Clinical Presentation

    1. Toxic effects mainly involve the cardiovascular system and the central nervous system (CNS).

TABLE 11-1 Classification of β-Blockers

Name	Adrenergic receptor antagonism	Partial agonist	Membrane stabilization	Lipid solubility	Oral bioavailability (%)	Vd (L/kg)	Elimination	Half-life (h)
Acebutolol	β_1	Yes	Yes	Moderate	40	2.3	Renal	3–6
Atenolol	β_1	No	No	Low	50	0.7	Renal	6–9
Betaxolol	β_1	No	Yes	Low	90	6.0	Hepatic	14–22
Bisoprolol	β_1	No	No	Low	80	2.7–3.1	Hepatic	9–12
Carteolol	β_1, β_2	No	No	Low	85	4.0	Renal	6
Carvedilol	β_1, β_2, α_1	Yes	No	High	25–35	1.6	Hepatic	6–10
Esmolol	β_1	No	No	Low	N/A	3.4	Esterase	0.15
Labetalol	β_1, β_2	Yes	No	Low	30–40	10	Hepatic	3–6
Metoprolol	β_1	No	No	Moderate–High	40–50	5.5	Hepatic	3–4
Nadolol	β_1, β_2	No	No	Low	30–50	2.1	Renal	14–24
Pindolol	β_1, β_2	Yes	Yes	Moderate	99	2.0	Renal	3–12
Propranolol	β_1, β_2	No	Yes	High	30	3.6	Hepatic	3–5
Sotalol	β_1, β_2	No	No	Low	90–100	0.2	Renal	5–12
Timolol	β_1, β_2	No	No	Low	75	1.5	Renal	4

2. Patients with severe toxicity typically develop hypotension and bradycardia.
   a. Cardioselectivity is often lost after overdose.
   b. Poisoning with agents possessing partial β receptor agonist activity (Table 11-1) can produce a normal or elevated heart rate.
3. Electrocardiogram (ECG) manifestations may include prolonged PR interval, intraventricular conduction delay, progressive atrioventricular block, nonspecific T-wave changes, early repolarization, and asystole.
4. Sotalol can cause ventricular tachycardia, including torsades de pointes, ventricular fibrillation, and multifocal ventricular extrasystoles.
5. CNS depression occurs with significant poisoning.
6. Seizures may develop, particularly after poisoning with lipophilic agents (e.g., propranolol, penbutolol, metoprolol).
7. Bronchospasm, a relatively rare consequence of β-blocker poisoning, usually occurs in patients with preexisting reactive airway disease.
8. Hypoglycemia is another infrequent complication of β-blocker toxicity. It appears to be more common in diabetics, children, and uremic patients and is caused by the blockade of hyperglycemic effects of catecholamines.

B. Evaluation
1. Evaluation should include cardiac monitoring, a 12-lead ECG and testing for serum electrolytes, glucose, blood urea nitrogen (BUN), creatinine, calcium, phosphorous, and magnesium.
2. Patients with severe poisoning should have a chest x-ray and arterial blood gas measurements taken. Invasive hemodynamic monitoring may also be helpful.

C. Differential Diagnosis
1. The differential diagnosis should include antidepressant, calcium channel blocker, clonidine, and digitalis poisoning.
2. Analphylactic, cardiogenic, septic, or hypovolemic shock should also be considered.

IV. TREATMENT

A. Advanced Life Support Measures should be instituted as necessary.
1. Consider early intubation for moderate to severely poisoned patients.
2. Begin with aggressive volume resuscitation for hypotension.

B. Decontamination (see Chapter 1)
1. Administer activated charcoal for recent overdose.
2. Consider multiple doses of activated charcoal for severely poisoned patients.
3. Consider whole bowel irrigation for overdoses of sustained-release preparations.

C. Pharmacologic Therapies
1. Multiple pharmacologic interventions are usually required for severely poisoned patients.

   2. Glucagon is the drug of choice for bradycardia and hypotension.
   a. It activates adenylate cyclase independent of the β receptor and is more effective than epinephrine or isoproterenol.
   b. Give a bolus dose of 5 to 10 mg intravenously (IV) (50 to 150 μg/kg IV for children), followed by continuous infusion of 1 to 10 mg/kg/hour (10 to 20 μg/kg/hour for children).
   3. Catecholamines may be effective, but large doses are often required and their proarrhythmic properties (particularly isoproterenol) limit their usefulness.
   4. Atropine is infrequently effective but has few contraindications.
   5. IV calcium, glucose–insulin–potassium therapy and a phosphodiesterase inhibitor such as milrinone should be considered for refractory cardiovascular depression (see Chapter 12).
   6. Hypertension and tachycardia from sotalol poisoning may be treated with short-acting agents such as nitroprusside and esmolol. Ventricular tachyarrhythmias should be treated with magnesium, lidocaine, phenytoin, or transvenous cardiac pacing (see Chapter 4).
   7. Seizures resulting from hypoglycemia should be treated with IV glucose. Those resulting from membrane effects should be treated with benzodiazepines or barbiturates.

D. Nonpharmacologic Therapy, such as transvenous cardiac pacing, intraaortic balloon pump counterpulsation, and cardiopulmonary bypass, should be considered for refractory cardiovascular depression.

V. COMPLICATIONS

A. Most patients recover fully if vital signs can be supported while the drug is endogenously metabolized and eliminated.

B. Although severe or prolonged shock can lead to myocardial infarction and multiple-organ failure, complete recovery has been reported even after cardiac arrest.

C. Aspiration pneumonia and sepsis can also occur.

Selected Readings
Adlerfliegel F, Leeman M, Demaeyer P, et al. Sotalol poisoning associated with asystole. *Intensive Care Med* 1993;19:57–58.
   A discussion of sotalol overdose.

Buiumsohn A, Eisenberg ES, Jacob H, et al. Seizures and intraventricular conduction defect in propranolol poisoning. *Ann Intern Med* 1979;91:860–862.
   A case report and discussion of propranolol.

Frishman W. Clinical pharmacology of the new beta-adrenergic blocking drugs. 1. Pharmacodynamic and pharmacokinetic properties. *Am Heart J* 1979;98:663–670.
   A discussion of β-blocking potency, cardioselectivity, partial agonist activity, membrane-stabilizing activity, and intrinsic sympathomimetic activity.

Frishman WH. Beta-adrenergic blockers. *Med Clin North Am* 1988;72:37–81.
   An extensive review of the pharmacology, indications, and adverse effects of β-blockers.

Gwinup GR. Propranolol toxicity presenting with early repolarization, ST changes and peaked T waves on EKG. *Ann Emerg Med* 1988;17:171–174.

A case report of an atypical presentation of propranolol toxicity with ST elevation, early repolarization, and peaked T waves (as opposed to the most common presentation of bradycardia and hypotension).

Hohnloser SH, Woosley Rl. Sotalol. *N Engl J Med* 1994;331:31–38.

A review article on sotalol, a β-adrenergic blocker, with a unique property of prolongation of the QT interval (class III antiarrhythmic).

Taboulet P, Cariou A, Berdeaux A, et al. Pathophysiology and management of self-poisoning with beta-blockers. *J Toxicol Clin Toxicol* 1993;31:531–551.

A review article containing an excellent overview of the pharmacologic management of β-blocker toxicity.

CALCIUM CHANNEL BLOCKERS
Steven B. Bird

12

I. BACKGROUND

A. Calcium channel blockers (CCBs) include a variety of agents that have antianginal, antiarrhythmic, and antihypertensive activity (Table 12-1).

B. Severe cardiovascular depression and myocardial ischemia can result from overdose.

II. PATHOPHYSIOLOGY

A. CCBs prevent extracellular calcium from entering into cardiac and smooth muscle through L-type, calcium-specific membrane channels.

    1. Mibefradil also blocks T-type calcium channels.

    2. Bepridil also has sodium-channel blocking activity.

B. Because calcium influx is necessary for muscle contraction, CCBs cause vasodilation, increase coronary blood flow, and decrease myocardial oxygen demand.

C. Verapamil and diltiazem also decrease sinus node discharge, conduction through the atrioventricular (AV) node, and cardiac contractility. Other CCBs do not appear to affect myocardial conduction and contractility at therapeutic doses.

D. Immediate-release preparations are well absorbed and have an onset of action within 30 minutes of ingestion.

E. Sustained-release preparations (available for diltiazem, nifedipine, and verapamil) have delayed onset and prolonged duration of toxicity in the overdose setting.

F. The smallest reported doses resulting in toxicity in adults are 720 mg for verapamil, 420 mg for diltiazem, and 50 mg for nifedipine.

III. DIAGNOSIS

A. Clinical Presentation

    1. Cardiovascular toxicity

        a. Hypotension and bradycardia are common. Hypotension can lead to myocardial ischemia and infarction.

        b. Verapamil and diltiazem can cause high-grade AV blockade or sinus arrest accompanied by a junctional escape rhythm.

        c. Poisoning by nifedipine and other vasodilators (Table 12-1) typically causes hypotension and tachycardia. Conduction disturbances are uncommon.

TABLE 12-1	Calcium Channel Blockers: Predominant Physiologic Effects

Negative chronotropic and inotropic effects
  Diltiazem
  Verapamil
Vasodilation
  Amlodipine
  Felodipine
  Israpadine
  Mibefradil
  Nicardipine
  Nifedipine
  Nimodipine
  Nisoldipine
Antianginal effects
  Bepridil
  Mibefradil
  Nifedipine

Source: Irwin RS, Rippe JM. *Irwin and Rippe's Intensive Care Medicine,* 5th ed. Philadelphia: Lippincott Williams & Wilkins, 2003:1416.

    d. Bepridil overdose can cause a prolonged QT interval and torsades de pointes.
  2. Noncardiac toxicity
    a. May include nausea, vomiting, lethargy, confusion, metabolic acidosis, noncardiogenic pulmonary edema, ileus, and mesenteric ischemia.
    b. Hyperglycemia may occur secondary to an inhibition of calcium-dependent insulin release.
    c. Seizures can occur after verapamil overdose.
  3. Chronic toxicity
    a. Occurs primarily in the elderly.
    b. Underlying liver disease and the combined use of other cardiac medications can exacerbate CCB toxicity.

B. Differential Diagnosis
  1. Other causes of hypotension and bradycardia include ischemic myocardial disease, stroke, hyperkalemia, and poisoning by antiarrhythmic agents, β-blockers, clonidine, digitalis, quinine, chloroquine, and tricyclic antidepressants.
  2. In contrast to CCB overdose, which can cause hyperglycemia, β-blocker poisoning is associated with hypoglycemia.

C. Evaluation
  1. Evaluation should include cardiac monitoring, a 12-lead electrocardiogram (ECG), and testing for serum electrolytes, glucose, blood urea nitrogen (BUN), creatinine, calcium, phosphorous, and magnesium.

2. Patients with severe poisoning should have a chest x-ray and arterial blood gas measurements taken. Invasive hemodynamic monitoring may also be helpful.

IV. TREATMENT

A. Advanced Life Support Measures should be instituted as necessary. Consider early intubation for severely poisoned patients.

B. Gastrointestinal Decontamination
   1. Activated charcoal should be considered for patients who present soon after acute overdose (see Chapter 1).
   2. Multiple-dose–activated charcoal and whole bowel irrigation should be considered for sustained-release preparation overdoses (see Chapter 1).

C. Hypotension and Bradycardia
   3. Hypotension should initially be treated with intravenous (IV) crystalloids.
   4. Severe cardiovascular toxicity generally does not respond to single-drug therapy and may require use of IV glucose–insulin–potassium, calcium, vasopressors, atropine, glucagon, and inamrinone.
      a. Glucose–insulin–potassium infusion
         (1) Also known as hyperinsulinemia/euglycemia (HIE) therapy.
         (2) Is superior to all other treatments in animal models and has been used successfully in humans.
         (3) Administer IV insulin bolus (1 to 2 IU/kg) followed by infusion (0.5 to 1.0 IU/kg/h) along with glucose (20% dextrose in water) and potassium to maintain euglycemia and normokalemia.
         (4) Serum glucose and potassium should be monitored frequently.
      b. Calcium
         (1) Variably effective in reversing hypotension but has minimal effect on bradycardia.
         (2) Give 1 to 2 g (10 to 20 mL of 10%) calcium chloride or 3 to 6 g (30 to 60 mL of 10%) calcium gluconate IV over 5 to 10 minutes.
         (3) Repeat bolus doses may be given every 5 to 10 minutes.
         (4) Large doses (10 g or more) may be required.
         (5) Monitor serum calcium and consider administration through a central venous line.
      c. Vasopressors (norepinephrine, epinephrine, dopamine) may be used to augment blood pressure, cardiac contractility, and heart rate.
      d. Atropine can be given for bradycardia and AV block but is not usually effective.
      e. Glucagon (see Chapter 11) can reverse myocardial depression as well as bradycardia.
      f. Inamrinone (formerly called amrinone)
         (1) Can be used to augment cardiac output.
         (2) Administer loading dose of 1 mg/kg followed by an infusion of 3 to 6 mg/kg/min.

   5. Intraaortic balloon pump or cardiac bypass pump support should be considered for patients with refractory hypotension.

D. Disposition
   (1) Asymptomatic patients presenting after an acute overdose of a non–sustained-release preparation require 4 to 6 hours of observation before medical clearance.
   (2) Patients with a sustained-release preparation overdose require 12 to 24 hours of observation.
   (3) All patients with hypotension, bradycardia, or AV block from CCBs require admission to an intensive care setting.

V. COMPLICATIONS

   A. Most patients recover fully if vital signs can be supported while the drug is endogenously metabolized and eliminated.
   B. Cerebral, myocardial, and mesenteric ischemia and infarction, multiple-organ failure, pneumonia, and sepsis can occur in patients with severe poisoning.

Selected Readings

Alousi AA, Canter JM, Fort DJ. The beneficial effect of amrinone on acute drug-induced heart failure in the anesthetized dog. *Cardiovasc Res* 1985;19:483–494.
This study demonstrated that amrinone improved myocardial contractility during calcium channel blocker toxicity.

Boyer EW, Shannon M. Treatment of calcium-channel-blocker intoxication with insulin infusion. *N Engl J Med* 2001;344:1721–1722.
Case series and description of hyperinsulinemia–euglycemia therapy.

Frierson J, Bailly D, Shultz T, et al. Refractory cardiogenic shock and complete heart block after unsuspected verapamil-SR and atenolol overdose. *Clin Cardiol* 1991; 14:933–935.
This case report showed the successful use of intraaortic balloon counterpulsation to improve cardiac output and blood pressure in the setting of a mixed calcium channel and β-adrenoreceptor blocker overdose.

Gay R, Angeo S, Lee R, et al. Treatment of verapamil toxicity in intact dogs. *J Clin Invest* 1986;77:1805–1811.
This study verified that increased serum calcium concentration improved inotropy and blood pressure in calcium channel blocker toxicity.

Kline JA, Leonva E, Raymond RM. Beneficial myocardial metabolic effects of insulin during verapamil toxicity in the anesthetized canine. *Crit Care Med* 1995; 23:1251–1263.
This study reported on high-dose insulin, showing improved survival when compared with calcium, epinephrine, or glucagon.

Ramoska EA, Spiller HA, Myers A. Calcium channel blocker toxicity. *Ann Emerg Med* 1990;19:649–653.
The limited efficacy of atropine alone in the treatment of bradycardia from calcium channel blocker toxicity was described in this article.

Ramoska EA, Spiller HA, Winter M, et al. A one-year evaluation of calcium channel blocker overdoses: toxicity and treatment. *Ann Emerg Med* 1993;22:196–200.
This analysis reported the various cardiac manifestations and treatments in patients with calcium channel blocker toxicity.

Roberts D, Honcharik N, Sitar DS, et al. Diltiazem overdose: pharmacokinetics of diltiazem and its metabolites and effect of multiple dose charcoal therapy. *J Toxicol Clin Toxicol* 1991;29:45–52.
This case report indicates that the beneficial effect of multiple-dose–activated charcoal therapy is not from enhancing serum drug clearance but to limiting further drug absorption.

Schoffstall JM, Spivey WH, Gambone JM, et al. Effects of calcium channel blocker overdose–induced toxicity in the conscious dog. *Ann Emerg Med* 1991; 20:1104–1108.
This study demonstrated the disparate hemodynamic effects of the calcium channel blocking agents in toxicity.

Tom PA, Morrow CT, Kelen GD. Delayed hypotension after overdose of sustained release verapamil. *J Emerg Med* 1994;12:621–625.
A case report demonstrating the markedly delayed onset of effects that may occur after the ingestion of sustained-release formulations of calcium channel blocking agents.

Wolf LR, Spadafora MP, Otten EJ. Use of amrinone and glucagon in a case of calcium channel blocker overdose. *Ann Emerg Med* 1993;22:1225–1228.
Amrinone was demonstrated to be successful in the management of calcium channel blocker poisoning in this case report.

Zaritsky AL, Horowitz M, Chernow B. Glucagon antagonism of calcium channel blocker–induced myocardial dysfunction. *Crit Care Med* 1988;16:246–251.
This study demonstrated that glucagon improved calcium channel blocker–induced myocardial depression.

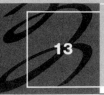

CHOLINERGIC AGENTS
Steven B. Bird

I. BACKGROUND

A. Causes of Cholinergic Poisoning
  1. Drugs that directly stimulate cholinergic receptors (e.g., bethanechol, pilocarpine, urecholine).
  2. Agents that inhibit acetylcholinesterase
      a. Organophosphate and carbamate insecticides
      b. Carbamate drugs (e.g., edrophonium, neostigmine, physostigmine, pyridostigmine, tacrine)
      c. Central acetylcholinesterase inhibitors (e.g., donepezil)
      d. Chemical warfare nerve agents such as GA (Tabun), GB (Sarin), GD (Soman), GF, and VX

B. Epidemiology
  1. Acute, severe, cholinergic poisoning is uncommon in the developed world.
  2. In developing countries, as many as 300,000 people die each year from ingestion of cholinergic insecticides.

II. PATHOPHYSIOLOGY

  A. The neurotransmitter acetylcholine and its muscarinic and nicotinic receptors are found in the central nervous system (CNS), including respiratory centers (muscarinic), the parasympathetic nervous system (muscarinic), sympathetic and parasympathetic ganglia (nicotinic), and the neuromuscular junction (nicotinic).
  B. Organophosphates can irreversibly inhibit acetylcholinesterase and cause toxicity lasting for days to months, until adequate amounts of the enzyme regenerate.
  C. Carbamates reversibly inhibit this enzyme and have a shorter duration of action.
  D. Effects of organophosphates and carbamates are predominantly caused by accumulation of acetylcholine at muscarinic and nicotinic synapses, resulting in sustained postsynaptic stimulation.
  E. Cholinergic agonists directly stimulate muscarinic receptors.

III. DIAGNOSIS

A. Clinical Presentation

1. Effects usually begin minutes to hours after dermal, pulmonary, or oral exposure.

2. Toxicity can be delayed with lipophilic organophosphates (e.g., fenthion, chlorfenthion) and those requiring hepatic metabolism to increase their toxicity (e.g., parathion).

3. Signs and symptoms of acetylcholinesterase inhibition can be divided into muscarinic, nicotinic, and CNS effects (Table 13-1). They are described by the mnemonics:

    a. DUMBELS (diarrhea, urination, miosis, bronchospasm/bronchorrhea, emesis, lacrimation, salivation) and

    b. SLUDGE (salivation, lacrimation, urination, defecation, gastric emesis).

4. Death usually results from respiratory failure, which is caused by central respiratory depression and diaphragmatic weakness.

B. Evaluation

1. Studies that should be obtained in symptomatic patients include electrocardiogram, arterial blood gases, chest x-ray, electrolytes, glucose, amylase, creatine kinase, and renal and liver function tests.

2. The severity of organophosphate poisoning correlates with the degree of depression of red blood cell (RBC) cholinesterase activity: mild (20% to 50% of baseline), moderate (10% to 20% of baseline), and severe (less than 10% of baseline).

    a. The diagnosis is usually confirmed retrospectively, because most facilities cannot measure cholinesterase enzyme activity on an immediate basis.

    b. Because of wide interindividual variability, significant depression of RBC cholinesterase activity can occur but still fall within the "normal" range.

TABLE 13-1	Signs and Symptoms of Cholinesterase Poisoning

Muscarinic	**Central nervous system**
Salivation	Respiratory depression
Lacrimation	Excitability
Bronchorrea/bronchoconstriction	Confusion
Urination	Agitation
Vomiting/diarrhea	Lethargy
Bradycardia	Coma
Miosis	Seizures
Nicotinic	Death
Muscle fasciculations	
Muscle weakness	
Muscle paralysis	
Tachycardia	
Hypertension	

3. Plasma ("pseudo") cholinesterase activity is a sensitive but less specific indicator of exposure; it can be depressed in a variety of medical conditions, including genetic deficiency.

IV. TREATMENT

A. Aggressive dermal and gastrointestinal decontamination (see Chapter 1) and supportive care with attention to adequate ventilation, prevention of aspiration, and control of respiratory secretions is essential.
B. Antidotal therapy
  1. Atropine
      a. Antagonizes acetylcholine only at muscarinic sites but is the primary treatment for serious cholinergic poisonings.
      b. Mildly symptomatic patients can be treated with usual doses.
      c. Treatment of severe poisoning should begin with an intravenous (IV) dose of 2 to 5 mg (0.05 mg/kg in children).
      d. Doses should be repeated or doubled every 3 to 5 minutes until signs of muscarinic excess abate.
          (1) Clearing of bronchial secretions and adequate oxygenation should be the therapeutic end points.
          (2) Pupillary dilatation and tachycardia are not reliable indications of adequate atropine therapy.
      e. Cumulative doses in the range of several hundred milligrams are not uncommon in severe organophosphate poisoning, and a continuous atropine drip may be easier to administer and titrate in this situation.
  2. Pralidoxime (2-PAM; Protopam)
      a. Reactivates acetylcholinesterase by reversing inhibitor binding and phosphorylation of the active site on this enzyme.
      b. Regenerates acetylcholinesterase at muscarinic, nicotinic, and CNS sites.
      c. Is indicated for nicotinic symptoms and moderate or severe clinical toxicity.
      d. Administer a loading dose of 25 to 50 mg/kg IV over 30 minutes. This dose can be repeated or followed by an infusion if signs of toxicity persist or recur.
      e. Continuous infusions (10 to 20 mg/kg/hour) offer improved kinetics over repeat bolus administration.
C. Diazepam should be used for the treatment of seizures.

V. COMPLICATIONS

A. Two types of delayed toxicity have been described in organophosphate poisoning.
  1. Intermediate syndrome
      a. Occurs 24 to 96 hours after the initial cholinergic crisis and may last 4 to 18 days.
      b. Characterized by paralysis of proximal limb muscles, neck flexor muscles, motor cranial nerves, and respiratory muscles in the absence of prominent muscarinic findings.

   c. May actually represent insufficient oxime therapy.
   d. Treatment is supportive and reinstitution of pralidoxime therapy.
2. Organophosphorus-induced delayed neurotoxicity (OPIDN)
   a. Peripheral neuropathy may develop 1 to 3 weeks after acute exposure to some organophosphorous agents.
   b. Appears to be mediated by "neurotoxic esterase" in peripheral neurons.
   c. May continue to worsen for several months, deficits may be permanent, and no specific therapy exists.

Selected Readings

Coye MJ, Barnett PG, Midtling JE, et al. Clinical confirmation of organophosphate poisoning by serial cholinesterase analyses. *Arch Intern Med* 1987;147:438–432.
A case series describing agricultural workers with organophosphate pesticide exposure that supports the use of sequential postexposure plasma cholinesterase analyses to confirm the diagnosis of organophosphate poisoning in the absence of baseline values.

Eddleston M, Phillips MR. Self poisoning with pesticides. *BMJ* 2004;328:42–44.
A review of the epidemic of developing world pesticide poisonings.

Eddleston M, Szinicz L, Eyer P, Buckley N. Oximes in acute organophosphorus pesticide poisoning: a systematic review of clinical trials. *QJM* 2002;95:275–283.
A thorough, critical review of the world's literature on oxime use.

Johnson MK. Organophosphates and delayed neuropathy—is NTE alive and well? *Toxicol Appl Pharmacol* 1990;102:385–399.
A review of the effects of organophosphates on neuropathy target esterase (NTE) and its relationship to polyneuropathy.

Lifshitz M, Rotenberg M, Sofer S, et al. Carbamate poisoning and oxime treatment in children: a clinical and laboratory study. *Pediatrics* 1994;93:652–655.
A retrospective series of children with carbamate poisoning demonstrates that oxime therapy will not exacerbate cholinergic symptoms.

Lotti M. Treatment of acute organophosphate poisoning. *Med J Aust* 1991;154:51–55.
This article reviews the methods of diagnosis and treatment of organophosphate and carbamate poisoning.

Lotti M, Becker CE, Aminoff MJ. Organophosphate polyneuropathy: pathogenesis and prevention. *Neurology* 1984;34:658–662.
This review describes the pathogenesis and clinical presentation of delayed organophosphate-induced polyneuropathy.

Senanayake N, Karalliedde L. Neurotoxic effects of organophosphorus insecticides: an intermediate syndrome. *N Engl J Med* 1987;316:761–763.
This report describes a characteristic constellation of delayed neurotoxic effects in patients with a particular organophosphate poisoning known as the intermediate syndrome.

Sidell FR, Borak J. Chemical warfare agents. II. Nerve agents. *Ann Emerg Med* 1992;21:865–871.
This review summarizes the clinical effects of nerve agent exposure and describes the management and treatment strategies for emergency medical personnel.

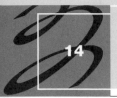

COCAINE POISONING
Ivan E. Liang

I. BACKGROUND

A. Illicit forms of cocaine include the hydrochloride salt and its alkalinization products, freebase and crack.

B. Cocaine hydrochloride is water-soluble, is readily absorbed through any mucosal surface, and can be administered intravenously (IV).

C. Freebase and crack are insoluble in water but can be smoked.

D. Oral overdose can occur in "body packers" (people who attempt to smuggle cocaine by ingesting wrapped and sealed packets of drug) and "body stuffers" (those who swallow or conceal loosely wrapped packets in body cavities when encountered by law enforcement agents) when packets rupture or leak.

II. PATHOGENESIS

A. Cocaine promotes the release of neurotransmitters (e.g., dopamine, norepinephrine) while also blocking their reuptake in the central and sympathetic nervous system.

B. Cocaine is also a local anesthetic that blocks initiation and conduction of nerve impulse by decreasing axonal membrane permeability to sodium ions; at high doses, this class I antiarrhythmic effect contributes to cardiotoxicity.

C. Cocaine is rapidly metabolized by liver esterases and plasma cholinesterase and by nonenzymatic hydrolysis. Only small amounts are eliminated as unchanged drug in urine. Patients with pseudocholinesterase deficiency may be at greater risk of toxicity because of their reduced capacity for metabolism through the pseudocholinesterase pathway.

D. After IV injection or inhalation, a subjective euphoric response occurs in 3 to 5 minutes, with a cardiovascular response peaking in 8 to 12 minutes and lasting approximately 30 minutes. After nasal insufflation (snorting) a euphoric effect occurs within 15 to 20 minutes, cardiovascular changes and plasma levels peak within 20 to 60 minutes, and effects last several hours. Time to onset, time to peak effect, and duration of effect are somewhat longer following ingestion. Effects can be markedly delayed and prolonged following packet ingestion.

III. CLINICAL PRESENTATION

A. Signs and symptoms of acute poisoning include elevated pulse, blood pressure, respirations, and temperature, the magnitude of which is roughly proportional to the degree of toxicity.

1. Patients with mild poisoning can have normal or nearly normal vital signs. Other manifestations include anxiety, agitation, euphoria, headache, tremors, twitching, nausea, vomiting, diaphoresis, mydriasis, and pallor.
2. Patients with moderate poisoning can manifest mild to moderately increased vital signs, confusion, hallucinations, hyperactivity, clonus, increased muscle tone, abdominal cramps, and brief tonic-clonic seizures. Tea-colored urine should alert the physician to the possibility of rhabdomyolysis and potential renal failure.
3. Patients with severe poisoning have markedly abnormal vital signs with malignant hyperthermia, tachydysrhythmias, and status epilepticus or coma with flaccid paralysis. Other manifestations include apnea, cyanosis, and Cheyne–Stokes respirations. Cardiovascular collapse, bradycardia, and hypotension are preterminal events.
4. Laboratory abnormalities include leukocytosis, hypokalemia, and hyperglycemia.
B. Chronic nasal use can result in rhinitis, epistaxis, and septal perforation. Systemic manifestations of chronic use include anorexia, weight loss, insomnia, formication, impotence, depression, paranoia, and psychosis.
C. Evaluation should focus on the cardiac, pulmonary, and neurologic systems. Continuous electrocardiographic (ECG) monitoring and frequent monitoring of vital signs, including core body temperature, are essential.
   1. Patients with moderate to severe toxicity should have the following: an ECG and chest x-ray study; analysis of complete blood count, electrolytes, glucose, blood urea nitrogen, creatinine, arterial blood gas, urinalysis, creatine, and phosphokinase; and qualitative toxicologic analysis of blood and urine.
   2. Finding cocaine and metabolites in the urine supports the diagnosis. However, because urine screening can detect cocaine metabolites for as long as 3 days after exposure, a positive screen does not equate with clinical toxicity.
   3. Standard protocols for ruling out myocardial infarction and ischemia should be followed in patients with chest pain of potential cardiac origin.
   4. Patients with a persistent or severe headache, abnormal neurologic examination, or prolonged seizures require computed tomography scan and lumbar puncture to rule out subarachnoid hemorrhage.
   5. Occult infections (e.g., endocarditis, hepatitis, pneumonia, epidural abscess) should be excluded in those with hyperthermia, particularly injection drug users.

IV. TREATMENT

A. Advanced life support measures should be instituted as necessary.
B. All patients should be closely observed, with IV access established and continuous ECG monitoring is necessary.
C. Supplemental oxygen, dextrose (25 g IV), and thiamine (100 mg IV) should be administered to patients with altered mental status, seizures, or coma.
D. Agitation, anxiety, and seizures can be treated with benzodiazepines (BZD), such as midazolam (2 to 5 mg IV), diazepam (2 to 10 mg IV), or lorazepam (1 to 4 mg IV).

E. Status epilepticus should be treated aggressively with IV BZD. Early paralysis and short-acting barbiturates (amobarbital, thiopental, pentobarbital) should be employed in refractory cases. Rocuronium (0.6 mg/kg) and vecuronium (0.08 to 0.1 mg/kg) are the preferred paralytic agents.

F. Paralysis, along with aggressive cooling measures, is also indicated in patients with severe hyperthermia.

G. Moderate hypertension and tachycardia usually respond to BZDs.

  1. Severe hypertension, particularly if associated with chest pain, is best treated with titratable IV agents, such as phentolamine (1 to 2 mg per dose), nitroglycerin, and nitroprusside.

  2. Phentolamine can be effective in reducing myocardial oxygen demand and improving coronary blood flow.

  3. β-adrenergic blocking agents (labetalol, esmolol, propranolol) are relatively contraindicated because they may worsen coronary vasospasm.

  4. Myocardial ischemia should otherwise be treated as usual. Adjunctive therapy with BZDs is recommended.

H. Dysrhythmias should be treated according to standard advanced cardiac life support (ACLS) protocols. Treatment of ventricular dysrhythmias should also include sodium bicarbonate (see Chapter 4).

I. Hypotension requires active fluid resuscitation. If vasopressor therapy is indicated, a direct-acting drug (e.g., norepinephrine) is preferred because cocaine depletes neurotransmitters and prevents their reuptake.

J. Gastrointestinal decontamination should include activated charcoal for recent ingestions (see Chapter 1).

K. Body packers or stuffers should be treated with multiple-dose charcoal plus laxatives or whole bowel irrigation (see Chapter 1).

  1. Endoscopic removal of intact packets must be performed with caution because packet rupture can occur.

  2. If signs or symptoms of cocaine toxicity are present or if intestinal obstruction occurs, immediate surgical intervention is indicated.

V. COMPLICATIONS

A. Complications can be acute or occur hours to days after actual cocaine use.

B. Cerebrovascular complications include cerebrovascular accidents, subarachnoid or intracerebral hemorrhage, and cerebral vasculitis.

C. Cardiovascular complications include myocardial, bowel, and kidney ischemia; myocardial infarction; skin necrosis; and aortic dissection.

D. Cerebral and renal vasculitis and cardiomyopathy have been reported.

E. Pulmonary infarcts, barotrauma, eosinophilia with granuloma formation, and noncardiogenic pulmonary edema can occur.

F. Inhalational exposure can result in cough, hemoptysis, reactive airway disease, pneumonitis ("crack lung"), and barotrauma (e.g., pneumothorax, pneumomediastinum).

Selected Readings

Gay GR, Inaba DS, Sheppard CW, et al. Cocaine: history, epidemiology, human pharmacology and treatment. A perspective on a new debut for an old girl. *Clin Toxicol* 1975;8:149–178.
Excellent discussion about historical usage of cocaine.

Hollander JE. The management of cocaine-associated myocardial ischemia. *N Engl J Med* 1995;333:1267–1272.
An excellent review article on the management of cocaine-associated chest pain.

Hollander JE, Hoffman RS. Cocaine-induced myocardial infarction: an analysis and review of the literature. *J Emerg Med* 1992;10:169–177.
Identification of a group of young individuals at risk for myocardial infarction.

Isner JM, Estes NA, Thompson PD, et al. Acute cardiac events temporally related to cocaine abuse. *N Engl J Med* 1986;315:1438–1443.
A report of seven patients with cardiac toxicity associated with nonintravenous use of cocaine.

Lange RA, Cigarroa RG, Flores ED, et al. Potentiation of cocaine-induced coronary vasoconstriction by β-adrenergic blockade. *Ann Intern Med* 1990;112:897–903.
Randomized, double-blind, placebo trial in cardiac catheterization laboratory showing effects of β-adrenergic blockade.

McCarron MM, Wood JD. The cocaine body packer syndrome. *JAMA* 1983;250:1417.
A prospective study of 75 body packers.

Mouhaffel AH, Madu EC, Satmary WA, et al. Cardiovascular complications of cocaine. *Chest* 1995;107:1426–1434.
A concise review of the cardiovascular complications of cocaine.

Pollack CV Jr, Biggers DW, Carlton FB Jr, et al. Two crack cocaine body stuffers. *Ann Emerg Med* 1992;21:1370–1380.
A discussion about the controversies regarding the management of cocaine body stuffers.

Roth D, Alarcon FJ, Fernandez JA, et al. Acute rhabdomyolysis associated with cocaine intoxication. *N Engl J Med* 1988;319:673–677.
A description of a group of cocaine-intoxicated patients with rhabdomyolysis and renal failure.

Spivey WH, Euerle B. Neurologic complications of cocaine abuse. *Ann Emerg Med* 1990;19:1422–1428.
A concise review of the neurologic complication of cocaine abuse.

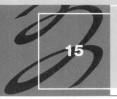

CORROSIVE INGESTIONS

Steven B. Bird

15

I. BACKGROUND

A. An acid is a substance that in aqueous solutions donates its proton or hydrogen (H^+) ion to a water molecule to form a hydronium ion, H_3O^+. An alkali is a substance in which hydroxyl (OH^-) ions are more prevalent than H^+ ions in aqueous solution.

B. Acids and alkalies are also known as caustics and corrosives.

C. Ingestion can result in respiratory distress as well as injury to the gastrointestinal (GI) tract.

D. The most commonly ingested alkaline substances are sodium and potassium hydroxide, sodium hypochlorite (bleach), sodium carbonate (washing soda or soda ash), sodium phosphate, sodium silicate, and ammonia. The most common acid ingestions include hydrochloric acid, sulfuric acid, boric acid, and phosphoric acid.

E. The severity of corrosive injury is related to many factors.

    1. Tissue toxicity is directly related to the titratable alkaline or acid reserve (TAR) of the ingested substance (i.e., the amount of acid or alkali needed to neutralize it to a pH of 7). The TAR reflects the pH (concentration) and volume of corrosive as well as its pKa (strength or intrinsic corrosivity).

        a. Greater tissue injury occurs at extremes of pH.

        b. Greater tissue injury occurs with a corrosive with a pKa less than 0 ("strong acids" such as nitric and sulfuric acid) or more than 14 ("strong bases" such as potassium and sodium hydroxide).

    2. Formulation

        a. Solids (powders and tablets) may adhere to tissue and thus have the greatest contact time, causing severe damage to the proximal gastrointestinal (GI) tract.

        b. Liquids are more likely to cause distal GI tract injury.

    3. Intent of exposure: Intentional exposures tend to involve larger volumes and have a greater propensity for serious injury than do accidental exposures.

    4. Stomach contents: Ingestions on an empty stomach, which provides no dilution or buffering effect, tend to be more severe than when the stomach is full.

    5. GI tract integrity: preexisting GI disorders may predispose an individual to corrosive injury.

II. PATHOPHYSIOLOGY

A. Acids cause coagulation necrosis as a result of protein denaturation. Subsequent eschar formation can potentially limit the depth of tissue penetration.

B. Alkalies cause liquefaction necrosis because of protein dissolution, collagen destruction, fat saponification, and cell membrane emulsification.

C. Deep tissue injury can result in perforation or scarring with strictures (especially with circumferential injuries).

III. DIAGNOSIS

A. Clinical Effects

1. Signs and symptoms can include oral burns (lips, tongue, oropharynx), epigastric pain, drooling, dysphagia, nausea, vomiting, hematemesis, coughing, choking, stridor, and respiratory distress.

2. The patient may also be asymptomatic at presentation.

3. Oropharyngeal burns correlate poorly with esophageal injury, and their absence does not rule out distal injury.

B. Evaluation

1. Evaluate the upper airway for patency.

2. Endoscopy is recommended for all symptomatic patients and those with large intentional ingestions.

a. Endoscopic visualization of the entire upper GI tract permits grading of the severity and extent of injury.

(1) A delay of 4 to 6 hours before endoscopy is recommended to avoid underestimating the severity of injury.

(2) Endoscopy should not be performed later than 24 hours after the ingestion to avoid iatrogenic perforation.

b. Endoscopy can be omitted:

(1) In pediatric patients with accidental ingestions and minimal symptoms who are able to swallow without difficulty.

(2) In patients with clinical or radiographic evidence of perforation or massive hemorrhage that will require surgical management.

c. If frank necrosis is encountered, evaluation of the more distal mucosa can be accomplished by percutaneous retrograde gastro-esophageal endoscopy or by laparotomy (indicated for possible or known perforation or massive hemorrhage).

d. Extent of mucosal injury is graded by the following:

(1) Grade I: erythema

(2) Grade IIa: superficial ulceration

(3) Grade IIb: deep or circumferential ulcerations

(4) Grade IIIa: small areas of necrosis

(5) Grade IIIb: extensive necrosis

3. Radiography

a. Contrast studies can be used to evaluate corrosive ingestions for perforation.

b. Staging of burn severity is not as accurate as endoscopy.

    c. Barium contrast esophagography may be useful after week 2 to evaluate for dysmotility or stricture formation.

C. Differential Diagnosis. The differential diagnosis of a corrosive injury includes anaphylaxis, angioedema, bowel perforation, esophageal foreign body or malignancy, infection (e.g., epiglottitis, Ludwig angina), thermal burns, and trauma (e.g., Boerhaave syndrome, iatrogenic esophageal injury).

IV. TREATMENT

A. Advanced Life Support Measures should be instituted as necessary.
    1. Perform immediate endotracheal intubation in patients with respiratory distress.
    2. Aggressive fluid resuscitation may be necessary in those with significant GI losses, bleeding, or tissue injury and consequent third spacing.

B. Gastrointestinal Decontamination
    1. Do not induce emesis or administer activated charcoal.
    2. Gastric lavage using a nasogastric tube should be considered for patients who present soon after liquid ingestions. Although of theoretical concern, there are no reported cases of iatrogenic perforation from gastric lavage.
    3. Dilution with water or milk may be beneficial immediately after ingestion. The ideal volume is unknown and care must be taken to avoid causing emesis.
    4. While some animal models support neutralizing an alkali with a weak acid (e.g., carbonated beverage, lemon juice) or an acid with a weak base (e.g., antacid), such therapy may theoretically result in additional heat or gas production and is controversial.
    5. All of these procedures are contraindicated if evidence of perforation exists.

C. Surgery
    1. Obtain emergency surgical consultation if signs of perforation, peritonitis, mediastinitis, or hemorrhage exist.
    2. Patients with grade III burns have a mortality rate of greater than 50% and a high rate of early complications and late sequelae, necessitating surgical intervention.

D. Prophylactic Corticosteroids (in conjunction with antibiotics) prevent stricture formation in experimental animals, but their efficacy in postexposure treatment remains controversial.
    1. Corticosteroids should be used for grade IIa or IIb esophageal burns only.
        a. Less severe injuries are unlikely to cause strictures.
        b. Most grade III or greater injuries develop strictures regardless of the use of steroids.

2. Methylprednisolone (40 mg IV every 8 hours in adults; 2 mg/kg/day divided three times a day in children) is given for 2 to 3 weeks, then tapered over 4 to 6 weeks.
3. Antibiotics (e.g., cefazolin, clindamycin) have a synergistic effect in experimental animals and should initially be given to all patients who receive corticosteroids.

E. **Other Agents** to consider include H$_2$–blockers, proton pump inhibitors, and sucralfate.

F. **Parenteral Alimentation** may be necessary in patients who are unable to eat. Resume enteral feeding as soon as tolerated.

V. COMPLICATIONS

A. Metabolic acidosis may result from large acid ingestions or extensive intestinal necrosis. Hemolysis, disseminated intravascular coagulation, and renal dysfunction have also been reported.
B. Various fistulae, including aortoesophageal, may develop subacutely or chronically.
C. Severely affected segments of esophagus may demonstrate partial or complete dysmotility. Strictures can occur as early as 2 weeks after ingestion.
D. Alkali injury increases the risk of squamous cell carcinoma of the esophagus (up to 40 times), with a latency period of decades.

Selected Readings

Broor SL, Kumar A, Chari ST, et al. Corrosive esophageal strictures following acid ingestion: Clinical profile and results of endoscopic dilation. *J Gastroenterol Hepatol* 1989;4:55–61.
A small longitudinal study showing that strictures after acid ingestions respond moderately well to endoscopic dilation but that recurrence of dysphagia is frequent and recurrent.

Byrne WJ. Foreign bodies, bezoars, and caustic ingestion. *Gastrointest Endosc Clin North Am* 1994;4:99–119.
An excellent review of the epidemiology, diagnosis, and acute and chronic treatment of pediatric caustic ingestions.

Gaudreault P, Parent M, McGuigan MA, et al. Predictability of esophageal injury from signs and symptoms: a study of caustic ingestion in 378 children. *Pediatrics* 1983;71:767–770.
A retrospective study of corrosive ingestions in 378 children under 14 years of age over a 10-year period. Ten patients had esophageal injuries of grade II, despite the absence of documented signs or symptoms.

Hawkins DB, Demeter MJ, Barnett TE. Caustic ingestion: controversies in management. A review of 214 cases. *Laryngoscope* 1980;90:98–109.
A review of 214 cases, including a 3-year prospective study of corticosteroid use. Four of five patients with moderately severe burns (now likely classified as grade IIb) did not develop strictures after steroid use, whereas seven of eight in the same group who did not receive steroids went on to develop strictures. No benefit was seen in the group with the most severe burns.

Howell JM, Dalsey WC, Hartsell FW, et al. Steroids for the treatment of corrosive esophageal injury: a statistical analysis of past studies. *Am J Emerg Med* 1992;10: 421–425.

A review of 361 corrosive ingestions. No patients with grade I burns developed strictures. Fifty-four of 228 patients (24%) with grade II or III burns developed strictures when steroids plus antibiotics were used, whereas 13 of 25 patients (52%) not treated with steroids despite grade II or III burns developed strictures.

Wu M-H, Lai W-W. Surgical management of extensive corrosive injuries of the alimentary tract. *Surg Gynecol Obstet* 1993;177:12–16.

A review of 28 patients taken for emergent laparotomy based on endoscopic findings of severe injury, peritoneal signs, or continuous GI bleeding. Overall mortality rate was 18%. The authors advocate aggressive surgical management for all severe corrosive ingestions.

Zargar SA, Kochnar R, Mehta S, et al. The role of fiberoptic endoscopy in the management of corrosive ingestion and modified endoscopic classification of burns. *Gastrointest Endosc* 1991;37:165–169.

A prospective study of 81 patients who underwent upper GI endoscopy after corrosive ingestion. No correlation between oropharyngeal burns and esophageal injury was found. No patients with burns of grade 0 to grade IIa developed strictures, 71% with grade IIb burns developed strictures, and all patients with grade III burns developed strictures (mean follow-up 24 months).

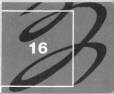

CYCLOSPORINE
Ivan E. Liang

16

I. BACKGROUND

A. Cyclosporine is an immunosuppressive drug, available orally (Neoral or Sandimmune) or intravenously (IV), that is used to prevent solid organ allograft rejection, graft-versus-host disease, and autoimmune diseases.

B. Toxicity can result from acute or chronic overdose.

II. PATHOPHYSIOLOGY

A. Cyclosporine blocks cytokine synthesis and receptor expression needed for T-lymphocyte activation. As a result, the activation and proliferation of helper and cytotoxic T cells, essential for the alloantigen rejection process, are disrupted.

B. Dose-related nephrotoxicity appears to result from interference of prostaglandin synthesis leading to intrarenal vasoconstriction. This may also be the cause of hypertension.

C. Hepatotoxicity is probably related to the inhibition of bile secretion pathways.

D. Cyclosporine is lipophilic and thus distributes widely throughout body tissues, concentrating in the liver, kidneys, and especially fat, producing higher cyclosporine concentrations than in the serum.

E. Peak serum levels occur 1 to 5 hours after therapeutic oral dosing. A redistribution phase lasts approximately 1.1 hours. Elimination half-life is 7 to 24 hours.

F. Oral cyclosporine undergoes extensive first-pass metabolism, which is why oral doses are considerably larger than IV doses.

G. Monitoring drug levels can prevent chronic toxicity. Trough concentrations (12 hours after the last dose) in whole blood (cyclosporine redistributes into erythrocytes) can be measured by a variety of assays (Table 16-1).

H. Drugs that induce or inhibit the hepatic cytochrome P-450 enzyme system can have significant effects on cyclosporine concentrations.

    1. Those that increase cyclosporine concentrations include ketoconazole, fluconazole, erythromycin, diltiazem, nicardipine, and cimetidine.

    2. Naringenin, a compound in grapefruit juice, causes an increase in both parent and metabolite cyclosporine levels by increasing its bioavailability.

TABLE 16-1		Cyclosporine 12-hour Trough Concentration Ranges for Various Analytic Methods	

Transplant	Sample matrix	Analytic method[a]	Target range (ng/mL)
Kidney	Blood	HPLC	150–250 (day 0–day 120) 100–200 (after day 120)
	Blood	P-FPIA or P-RIA[b]	200–800
	Blood	M-RIA or M-FPIA	150–400
	Serum/plasma	P-FPIA	100–250
Liver	Blood	HPLC	150–300
		M-RIA or M-FPIA	150–400
		P-FPIA	400–800
Heart	Blood	HPLC	150–300
		M-RIA or M-FPIA	150–400
Bone marrow	Serum/plasma	P-FPIA or P-RIA[b]	100–250

Source: Irwin RS, Rippe JM. *Manual of Intensive Care Medicine,* 3rd ed. Philadelphia: Lippincott Williams & Wilkins, 2000:625.
[a]HPLC, high-performance liquid chromatography; M-RIA monoclonal radioimmunoassay; M-FPIA, monoclonal fluorescence polarization immunoassay; P-FPIA, polyclonal fluorescence polarization immunoassay; P-RIA, polyclonal radioimmunoassay.
[b]No longer available.

III. DIAGNOSIS

A. Clinical Toxicity

1. The most common signs and symptoms after intentional and therapeutic overdoses are hypertension, tachycardia, tremor, nausea and vomiting, and drowsiness.
2. Gingivitis, gastric discomfort, hepatotoxicity (transaminase and bilirubin elevations), renal insufficiency (rising creatinine level), and burning sensations in the mouth, feet, and face have also been reported.
3. Neurotoxicity (encephalopathy, seizures, headache, visual disorders, white-matter changes, and coma) can occur in patients with very high blood concentrations, low cholesterol and magnesium levels as well as in liver transplant recipients.
4. Oliguric renal failure, metabolic acidosis, and respiratory depression have also been reported, particularly in the pediatric population.

B. Evaluation

1. Laboratories studies should include complete blood count (CBC), electrolytes, blood urea nitrogen (BUN), creatinine, glucose, liver functions tests, and cyclosporine level.
2. Evaluation of intentional overdoses should include an electrocardiogram (ECG) and serum acetaminophen and salicylate levels.
3. Cyclosporine levels may not correlate with clinical toxicity following acute overdose.

IV. TREATMENT

A. Advanced life support measures and supportive care should be instituted as necessary.

B. In patients on chronic therapy, cyclosporine should be discontinued until drug levels are in the therapeutic range.

C. For persisting or worsening renal failure, consultation with a nephrologist is warranted.

D. Seizures should be treated with benzodiazepines.

E. Activated charcoal should be considered for recent acute overdose (see Chapter 1).

F. Hemodialysis and hemoperfusion are not likely to be of benefit because of cyclosporine's high volume of distribution.

G. Exchange transfusion has been used for neonatal overdose but is of unclear benefit.

V. COMPLICATIONS: Although toxicity typically resolves with decreasing drug levels, chronic renal insufficiency can occur.

Selected Readings

Arellano F, Monka C, Krupp PF. Acute cyclosporin overdose. A review of present clinical experience. [Published erratum appears in *Drug Saf* 1991;6:338.] *Drug Saf* 1991;6:266–276.
Summary of toxic effects on 27 patients with oral or parenteral overdosage of cyclosporine and suggested guidelines for management.

de Groen PC, Aksamit AJ, Rakela J, et al. Central nervous system toxicity after liver transplantation: the role of cyclosporine and cholesterol. *N Engl J Med* 1987; 317:861–866.
A case series of patients with cyclosporine-associated central nervous system toxicity associated with low cholesterol levels.

Honcharik N, Anthone S. Activated charcoal in acute cyclosporin overdose. *Lancet* 1985;1:1051.
A case report describing the effects of activated charcoal on acute oral cyclosporine overdose.

Kahan BD. Cyclosporine. *N Engl J Med* 1989;321:1725–1738.
A comprehensive review of cyclosporine, including pharmacology and toxic effects.

Kokado Y, Takahara S, Ishibashi M, et al. An acute overdose of cyclosporine. *Transplantation* 1989;47:1096–1097.
A case report describing the hepatotoxic effects of an acute oral overdose of cyclosporine.

Ptachcinski RJ, Venkataramanan R, Burckart GJ. Clinical pharmacokinetics of cyclosporin. *Clin Pharmacokinet* 1986;11:107–132.
A detailed review of the pharmacology and therapeutic monitoring of cyclosporine.

Rush DN. Cyclosporine toxicity to organs other than the kidney. *Clin Biochem* 1991;24:101–105.
A detailed review of cyclosporine toxicity to multiple organs.

Thompson CB, June CH, Sullivan KM, et al. Association between cyclosporin neurotoxicity and hypomagnesaemia. *Lancet* 1984;2:1116–1120.
A case series of bone-marrow transplant recipients with cyclosporine neurotoxicity associated with hypomagnesemia.

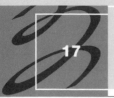

17

DIGITALIS
Steven B. Bird

I. BACKGROUND

- **A.** Digitalis, an extract from *Digitalis purpurea* (purple foxglove), contains digoxin and other steroid glycosides that have been used in the treatment of heart failure for more than 200 years.
- **B.** Similar cardiac glycosides are found in other plants (e.g., dogbane, *Nerium* spp, lily of the valley, red squill or *Urginea maritima*) and in the skin secretions of *Bufo* toad species.
- **C.** Manifestations of cardiac glycoside poisoning include gastrointestinal (GI), cardiac, central nervous system, and visual effects.

II. PATHOPHYSIOLOGY

- **A.** Cardiac glycosides inhibit the sodium–potassium adenosine triphosphatase (Na-K-ATPase) pump, resulting in changes in intracellular sodium and calcium, decreased atrial and atrioventricular (AV) nodal conduction velocity, and enhanced cardiac contractility.
- **B.** Toxic cardiac effects include increased vagal tone, AV block, and increased automaticity.
- **C.** Therapeutic serum digoxin levels are 0.8 to 2.0 ng/mL.
  - **1.** Absorption and distribution are slow.
  - **2.** Serum drug levels obtained before distribution is complete (within 6 hours of administration) will be higher than tissue levels and will not correlate with effect.
- **D.** Digoxin is primarily eliminated by renal excretion; clearance is reduced in renal failure, resulting in increased serum concentrations.
- **E.** Increased sensitivity to the effects of cardiac glycosides is seen in the elderly and in patients with cardiomyopathy, myocardial ischemia, electrolyte disturbances (hypokalemia, hypomagnesemia, and hypercalcemia), renal dysfunction, hepatic disease, hypothyroidism, and chronic obstructive pulmonary disease.
- **F.** Increased digoxin levels or effect can result from concomitant therapy with amiodarone, cyclosporine, erythromycin, neomycin, propafenone, quinidine, tetracycline, and verapamil.

III. DIAGNOSIS

A. Clinical Toxicity
  - **1.** GI symptoms include anorexia, nausea, vomiting, and abdominal pain.
  - **2.** Cardiac manifestations are common and frequently life-threatening.

    a. Arrhythmias frequently associated with cardiac glucoside toxicity include:

      (1) ventricular premature beats

      (2) supraventricular tachycardia with a conduction block

      (3) junctional tachycardia

      (4) sinus bradycardia

      (5) AV nodal blocks

      (6) ventricular tachycardia

      (7) ventricular fibrillation

    b. Tachycardia (enhanced automaticity) with variable AV block (impaired conduction), accelerated junctional rhythm (regularization of atrial fibrillation), and fascicular tachycardia are highly suggestive of cardiac glucoside toxicity.

  3. Neuropsychiatric manifestations include confusion, delirium, depression, hallucinations, headache, lethargy, vertigo, and seizures.

  4. Visual changes include cloudy, blurred, and diminished vision and yellow-green halos or images appearing washed in yellow (xanthopsia).

  5. General complaints such as fatigue, weakness, and dizziness are also common.

  6. Acute poisoning of the Na-K-ATPase pump can result in markedly elevated serum potassium levels.

    a. A serum potassium concentration of more than 5.5 mEq/L is predictive of mortality after acute digoxin overdose.

    b. In contrast, hypokalemia and hypomagnesemia are commonly seen in chronic intoxication.

  7. Chronic intoxication may be subtle and mimic common illnesses such as influenza or gastroenteritis.

B. Evaluation

  1. All patients should have continuous cardiac monitoring and an electrocardiogram.

  2. Ancillary testing should include evaluation of serum electrolytes, calcium, and magnesium; renal function tests; oxygen saturation or arterial blood gas analysis; a serum digoxin concentration; and a chest radiograph.

    a. Serial serum digoxin and potassium concentrations should be obtained, particularly following acute overdose.

    b. Drug levels should be interpreted with respect to time since last dose and in the overall clinical context and not relied on as the sole indicator of the presence or absence of toxicity.

    c. An elevated digoxin concentration supports the diagnosis. However, some patients develop toxicity at therapeutic concentrations, and others can be asymptomatic despite toxic concentrations.

IV. TREATMENT

  A. Advanced life support measures should be instituted as necessary. Meticulous attention to supportive care and a search for correctable conditions (e.g., hypoxia, hypoventilation, hypovolemia, hypoglycemia, electrolyte disturbances) are essential.

B. Activated charcoal should be considered in patients with recent ingestions (see Chapter 1).

    1. If gastric intubation is performed, pretreatment with atropine is recommended because this procedure can cause vagal stimulation and bradycardia.

    2. Multiple doses of activated charcoal (see Chapter 1) should be administered to enhance the elimination of digoxin.

C. Atropine is the initial therapy for bradycardia and AV block resulting in hypotension or worsening heart failure.

    1. Because of concerns about pacer-induced ventricular fibrillation, antidotal therapy with digoxin-specific antibody Fab fragments (Digibind or DigiTab) is recommended for symptomatic bradydysrhythmias that are unresponsive to atropine.

    2. Asymptomatic bradydysrhythmias do not require treatment.

D. Fab fragments are also the treatment of choice for potentially life-threatening ventricular tachyarrhythmias, other conduction disturbances, and myocardial depression.

E. Antiarrhythmic therapy is recommended as a temporizing measure for ventricular tachyarrhythmias.

    1. Phenytoin has classically been the antiarrhythmic of choice because it increases the ventricular fibrillation threshold and enhances conduction through the AV node.

    2. Intravenous magnesium (2 to 4 g IV over 1 min) has been effective in counteracting ventricular irritability.

    3. Lidocaine is also acceptable but not often effective.

F. Electrical cardioversion can precipitate ventricular fibrillation and should be performed with extreme caution; a low energy setting should be used.

G. Supplemental potassium may be beneficial in chronic digitalis toxicity when diuretic-induced hypokalemia is a factor.

H. Potassium should not be routinely administered to the acutely poisoned patient because hyperkalemia may ensue.

    1. Fab fragments are the treatment of choice for patients with hyperkalemia secondary to acute intoxication.

    2. Hyperkalemia can also be treated with IV glucose, insulin, and sodium bicarbonate.

    3. Calcium may enhance digitalis cardiac toxicity and should be avoided.

I. The dose of Fab fragment is based on the estimated body load of digoxin.

    1. The body load is equal to the amount (mg) of an acute ingestion or, in chronic intoxication, the serum digoxin level (ng/mL) multiplied by 5.6 times the body weight (kg) and divided by 1,000.

    2. One vial of Fab (40 mg) will bind 0.6 mg of digoxin. The number of vials required can be calculated by dividing the total body burden by 0.6.

    3. Patients with acute digoxin poisoning have a much higher body load than those with chronic poisoning.

        a. If the amount of an acute ingestion is unknown, empiric therapy should begin with five to ten vials.

        b. If the serum level is not known, empiric therapy should begin with one to two vials in patients with chronic intoxication.

        c. Similar empiric therapy can be used for other cardiac glucoside exposures.

4. If cardiac arrest is imminent or has occurred, the dose can be given as a bolus. Otherwise, it should be infused over 30 minutes.

J. A precipitous drop in serum potassium, the emergence of supraventricular tachydysrhythmias previously controlled by digoxin, and worsening of congestive heart failure in a patient dependent on digoxin for inotropic support are potential complications of Fab fragment therapy. Allergic reactions are rare and can be treated with standard measures.

K. After administration of Fab fragments, the serum digoxin concentration will increase dramatically owing to redistribution into the blood. Therefore, unless free drug levels can be obtained, measuring the digoxin concentration after Fab therapy is not useful.

V. COMPLICATIONS

A. Multiple-organ failure may result from inadequate tissue perfusion secondary to dysrhythmias or cardiovascular depression.

B. Recurrence of toxicity days after Fab fragment treatment is possible in functionally anephric patients who are unable to excrete the antibody–digoxin complex.

Selected Readings

Antman EM, Wenger TL, Butler VP, et al. Treatment of 150 cases of life-threatening digitalis intoxication with digoxin-specific Fab antibody fragments: final report of a multi-center study. *Circulation* 1990;81:1744–1752.
A multicenter study of Fab fragment in which 90% of patients had a treatment response.

Bismuth C, Gaultier M, Conso F, et al. Hyperkalemia in acute digitalis poisoning: prognostic significance and therapeutic implications. *Clin Toxicol* 1973;153:153–162.
A study demonstrating the prognostic importance of hyperkalemia. Patients with potassium above 5.5 mEq/L had 100% mortality.

Eddleston M, Rajapakse S. Rajakanthan K, et al. Anti-digoxin Fab fragments in cardiotoxicity induced by ingestion of yellow oleander: a randomised controlled trial. *Lancet* 2000;355:967–972.
A randomized controlled trial demonstrating the efficacy of digoxin Fab in the treatment of acute oleander digitalis glycoside poisoning.

Fisch C, Knoehel SB. Digitalis cardiotoxicity. *J Am Coll Cardiol* 1985;5:91A–98A.
Excellent review of the most electrophysiologic mechanism for digitalis-induced arrhythmias.

Ingelfinger JA, Goldman P. The serum digitalis concentration—does it diagnose digitalis toxicity? *N Engl J Med* 1976;294:867–870.
A discussion of the importance and limitations of serum digitalis levels and the significance of clinical information such as renal function, serum potassium, and cardiac impairment in the diagnosis of digitalis toxicity.

Kelly RA, Smith TW. Recognition and management of digitalis toxicity. *Am J Cardiol* 1992;69:108G–118G.
A discussion of the recognition and management of the factors leading to increased risk of toxicity in certain patients.

Lewis RP. Clinical use of serum digoxin concentrations. *Am J Cardiol* 1992:69: 97G–106G.
A discussion of the use and limitations of digoxin concentrations as well as the technical problem with the serum assay.

Smith TW. Digitalis: mechanisms of action and clinical use. *N Engl J Med* 1988;318: 358–365.
An excellent discussion about sodium and calcium effects on the excitation–contraction coupling and the mechanism of action of digitalis.

Taboulet P, Baud FJ, Bismuth C, et al. Acute digitalis intoxication—is pacing still appropriate? *J Toxicol Clin Toxicol* 1993;31:261–273.
A retrospective study comparing the outcome of cardiac pacing versus Fab fragments. Results favor fragments, but they are not statistically significant.

Woolf AD, Wenger T, Smith TW, et al. The use of digoxin-specific Fab fragments for severe digitalis intoxication in children. *N Engl J Med* 1992;326:1739–1744.
Recommendation for the use of Fab fragments based on its use in 29 children and adolescents. Data support the idea that adolescents are more sensitive to the effects of digitalis than younger children are.

Ivan E. Liang

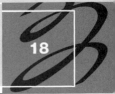

I. CROTALINE SNAKE ENVENOMATION

A. Background

1. Members of the Crotilinae genera include *Crotalus* (rattlesnakes) and *Agkistrodon* (copperheads and water moccasins or cottonmouths).
2. These snakes typically have elliptical pupils and temperature-sensing pits just in front of the eyes (hence the common name "pit viper").
3. Several thousand envenomations occur in the United States each year, but deaths are rare. Up to 25% of bites are "dry" (without envenomation).
4. Information regarding exotic (imported) snake envenomation can be obtained from zoos and regional Poison Centers (800-222-1222).

B. Pathophysiology

1. Crotaline snake venom comprises a complex mixture of necrotic and hemotoxic components, capable of causing both local and systemic injury.
2. The Mojave rattlesnake (*Crotalus scutulatus scutulatus*) is an exception; its venom contains neurotoxins.

C. Diagnosis

1. Clinical manifestations
   a. Dry bites should produce no signs or symptoms other than those of a puncture wound. A component of anxiety may complicate this diagnosis.
   b. Signs and symptoms of envenomation are usually apparent within minutes to a few hours but can be delayed for up to 12 hours.
      (1) Local effects
         i. Within minutes, stinging and burning pain begins.
         ii. Progressive swelling, erythema, petechiae, ecchymosis, and hemorrhagic blistering may occur.
         iii. Tissue edema and necrosis can result in compartment syndromes.
      (2) Systemic effects
         i. Typically include nausea, vomiting, weakness, muscle fasciculations, parasthesias (perioral and peripheral).
         ii. Coagulopathy, particularly thrombocytopenia and fibrinolysis, may occur.
         iii. Anemia, hemolysis, rhabdomyolysis, and cardiovascular collapse can result from severe envenomations.
      (3) Copperhead envenomation is often limited to local effects.

(4) Mojave rattlesnake envenomation often resembles that from Elapidae, with minimal local effects and delayed (by several hours) neurologic signs including muscle weakness, ptosis, and even diaphragmatic weakness.

(5) More severe effects occur in patients with extremes of age, delayed presentation, and more centrally located envenomations.

2. Evaluation
   a. There are no specific tests that can confirm or exclude envenomation. The diagnosis is based on the history and clinical findings.
   b. Envenomation can be ruled out only by prolonged observation.
   c. Local edema should be followed closely by serial evaluations (circumference measurements in affected extremities).
   d. Patients with massive edema or signs of limb ischemia should have intracompartmental pressure measurements taken.
   e. Patients with signs or symptoms of envenomation should have complete blood count (CBC), coagulation profile, electrolytes, blood urea nitrogen (BUN), and creatinine tested.
   f. In severe cases, creatine kinase, fibrinogen, fibrin split products, and arterial blood gases should be measured.

3. Differential diagnosis: Snakebite may be misdiagnosed as a venomous or nonvenemous arthropod or reptile bite or sting, as a wound from thorns or brush, or as an allergic reaction or infection.

D. Management

1. Advanced life support measures should be provided as needed.
   a. Endotracheal intubation may be necessary for airway protection in patients with facial envenomations.
   b. IV fluids should be given for hypotension.

2. Local wound care should be instituted, with tetanus prophylaxis if necessary and antibiotics for evidence of infection.
   a. Constricting clothing and jewelry should be removed and an affected limb immobilized at the level of the heart.
   b. Use of tourniquet or suction devices is not recommended.

3. Systemic effects should be treated with antivenom and supportive care.
   a. Minimal indications for antivenom include marked swelling, severe pain, and presence of fang marks.
   b. Prompt treatment is indicated for progressive swelling or any systemic signs (fasciculations, coagulopathy, muscle weakness).
   c. Suspected Mojave rattlesnake envenomation remains controversial owing to the lack of immediate and local symptoms.
   d. Two types of antivenoms are available:
      (1) The older Crotalinae polyvalent (equine-derived) antivenom has become less favored because it often retains residual equine serum components and has a higher incidence of allergic reactions.
      (2) The newer Crotalinae polyvalent Fab is ovine derived and composed of nearly pure Fab fragments.
   e. Relative contraindications are known hypersensitivity to the antivenom, to horse or sheep serum, or to papain or papayas (used to derive the Fab antivenom). A horse serum test kit is included with equine-derived antivenom. Skin testing is controversial and should be

done only if antivenom treatment is imminent. Epinephrine and diphenhydramine should be available at the bedside.

   f. Equine polyvalent antivenom should be given initially as 5 vials for mild envenomations (local pain and swelling), 10 vials for moderate (progressive swelling, ecchymosis, mild systemic symptoms), and 15 vials for severe (rapidly progressive swelling, hypotension, coagulopathy).

   g. Fab antivenom should be given initially as four vials for mild envenomations, six vials for moderate, and eight vials for severe.

   h. Fab antivenom routinely requires multiple dosing because of its short half-life; the package insert recommends consideration of two-vial redosing every 6 hours for three additional doses in severe envenomations.

   i. Treatment with equine polyvalent antivenom is usually associated with serum sickness. Very rarely, it may occur with the Fab antivenom. Onset of mild fevers, myalgias, and rash typically occur 5 to 14 days after administration and can usually be managed with supportive care and corticosteroids, antiinflammatories, and antihistamines.

  4. Coagulopathy may not respond to antivenom therapy, but bleeding is uncommon and treatment with fresh-frozen plasma (or other blood products) is rarely necessary.

E. Complications

  1. Edema typically resolves without sequelae. Fasciotomy should not be undertaken without documenting elevated compartment pressures and failure to respond to antivenom.

  2. Rhabdomyolysis should be treated with IV fluids and bicarbonate.

II. ELAPIDAE ENVENOMATION

A. Background

  1. Coral snakes, the only members of the Elapidae family indigenous to North America, include the Eastern coral snake (*Micrurus fulvius fulvius*), the Texas coral snake (*Micrurus fulvius tenere*), and the Arizona (Sonoran) coral snake (*Micruroides euryxanthus*).

  2. Elapids lack heat-sensing pits and have round pupils. Their fangs are small and often require the snake to "chew" its victim for significant envenomations.

  3. They are brightly colored and generally nonaggressive. Typical coloration is a red band next to a yellow band, hence the phrase: "Red on yellow, kill a fellow; red on black, venom lack."

B. Pathophysiology. Elapid snake venom contains predominantly neurotoxins.

C. Diagnosis

  1. Clinical manifestations

   a. Local effects are typically minimal and may include minor pain without evidence of inflammation or swelling.

   b. Systemic symptoms are often delayed so prolonged observation is mandatory (12 to 24 hours for suspected envenomation).

   c. Symptoms may start with numbness and weakness and may progress to drowsiness, apprehension, fasciculation, tremors, difficulty swallowing, dyspnea, salivation, nausea, and vomiting.

   d. Other findings may include weakness of extraocular muscles, miotic pupils, bulbar paralysis, ptosis, respiratory depression, and convulsions.

2. Evaluation

   a. There are no specific tests that can confirm or exclude envenomation. The diagnosis is based on the history and clinical findings.

   b. Routine laboratory tests should be obtained as clinically indicated.

   c. Pulmonary function tests (e.g., forced vital capacity) and arterial blood gas measurement may be helpful in assessing respiratory function.

3. Differential diagnosis

   a. The diagnosis is usually straightforward because it typically involves a brightly colored snake latching onto the victim.

   b. Late presentations in which the patient has difficulty communicating may be confused with botulism and motor neuron diseases, although the progression is typically more rapid with elapid envenomation than with other conditions.

D. Management

1. Advanced life support measures should be provided as needed. Endotracheal intubation may be necessary for patients with bulbar paralysis, dysphagia, or respiratory failure.

2. Wound care is the same as that for crotaline snakebites.

3. Systemic effects can be successfully treated with supportive care alone, but antivenom can prevent progression to airway compromise and ventilatory failure if delivered in a timely manner.

   a. Because late administration of antivenom may not reverse existing toxicity, at least five vials of *M. fulvius* antivenom (equine) should be given by IV infusion to any patient who has clearly been bitten by an elapid or who develops systemic signs and symptoms.

   b. Redosing may be necessary if symptoms progress.

   c. *M. fulvius* antivenom is prepared similarly to crotalid equine antivenom and carries the same risks of hypersensitivity and serum sickness (see earlier).

4. All patients with potential elapid envenomation should be admitted for serial examinations.

E. Complications

1. Neuromuscular dysfunction typically resolves without sequelae.

2. As with crotaline antivenom, patients who receive *M. fulvius* antivenom will likely develop serum sickness. The time course and treatment are the same.

III. BLACK WIDOW SPIDER ENVENOMATION

A. Background

1. *Lactrodectus* species (black widow spiders, or BWSs), predominantly *L. mactans* and *L. hesperus,* are found throughout most of the continental United States.

2. They are typically 1 to 2 cm in size and have a shiny black body with a red violin-shaped marking on the ventral abdomen. Venom is injected through hollow fangs.

3. BWSs usually live in relatively undisturbed locations near human habitation, such as outhouses, wood piles, and garages.

4. Although envenomation can be extremely painful, life-threatening effects are very rare.

B. Pathophysiology

1. *Latrodectus* venom contains α-latrotoxin, which promotes the release of norepinephrine from adrenergic neurons, acetycholine from cholinergic neurons, and catecholamines from adrenal glands.

2. Muscle cramping (resulting from motor endplate acetylcholine release) is thought to be the cause of pain.

C. Diagnosis

1. Clinical presentation

  a. Black widow spider bite is typically described as a sharp pinprick, but it is often unrecognized.

  b. A characteristic target lesion (a 2 to 6 cm erythematous ring with central pallor) develops at the site of a bite in 2 to 24 hours.

  c. Localized and then diffuse pain, muscle cramps (typically of the abdomen or back), tachycardia, and hypertension appear within 30 to 120 minutes.

  d. Diaphoresis and piloerection, sometimes isolated to the bite site, can occur.

  e. Rarely reported effects include periorbital edema and ecchymosis, priapism, cardiac dysrhythmias (including reflex bradycardia), and paralysis.

  f. Young children may simply present with inconsolable crying or restlessness.

  g. Although symptoms usually peak within several hours and, if untreated, wane over several days, they can be delayed for up to 24 hours and can last for months.

  h. The catecholamine effect can compromise patients at age extremes and those with significant, underlying cardiopulmonary disease.

  i. Pregnant patients may develop uterine contractions and a preeclampsia-like state, but there are no reported cases of fetal complications.

2. Evaluation

  a. There are no specific tests that can confirm or exclude envenomation. The diagnosis is based on the history and clinical findings.

  b. Routine laboratory studies should include CBC, electrolytes, BUN, and creatinine. Creatine phosphokinase should be obtained to check for possible rhabdomyolysis.

3. Differential diagnosis

  a. The pain from BWS envenomation may be confused with that from a broad variety of causes, including acute abdominal conditions (perforated viscous, appendicitis, and nephrolithiasis; envenomated patients have erroneously gone on to surgical exploration) as well as musculoskeletal disorders and scorpion envenomation.

    b. Typically, patients with BWS envenomation lie still between episodes of muscle contraction, which may help distinguish it from other conditions.

D. Treatment

1. Wound care is the same as for crotaline snakebites.
2. Asymptomatic patients should be observed for 6 hours.
3. Mild pain can often be controlled with oral opiates.
4. Moderate and severe pain should be treated with IV opiates and benzodiazepines.
5. Equine-derived BWS antivenom should be reserved for patients who do not respond to opiates and benzodiazepines.

   a. That available in the United States is targeted to *L. mactans* but is effective for all North American species.

   b. It carries the same risks of hypersensitivity and serum sickness as crotaline snake equine antivenom (see earlier).

   c. In most cases, a single IV dose (vial) will relieve symptoms within 30 min to 1 hour.

E. Complications

1. Symptoms resolve without sequelae. Significant pain in patients not treated with antivenom typically lasts several days, but minor muscle aches may persist for up to a month.
2. Serum sickness in those who receive antivenom is less likely than with snake envenomation because smaller quantities of antivenom are administered. The time course and treatment are the same.

IV. BROWN RECLUSE SPIDER ENVENOMATION

A. Background

1. *Loxosceles reclusa* (brown recluse spider, or BRS), the most common spider of this genus in the United States, is found in the southern Midwestern states (outdoors or indoors), but other *Loxosceles* species are found worldwide.
2. The BRS typically measures 1 to 5 cm from leg to leg, has a light or dark brown short-haired body with slender legs, and has a violin-shaped dark brown marking on its dorsal cephalothorax.
3. The BRS is reclusive and typically avoids human contact and activity.

B. Pathophysiology

1. BRS venom consists of a mixture of mostly cytotoxic components (e.g., protease, S-ribonucleotide phosphohydrolase, hyaluronidase, collagenase, esterase, sphingomyelinase-D).
2. The classic dermonecrotic lesion results from endothelial cell damage by venom and ischemia secondary to inflammation caused by leukocyte infiltration, hemolysis, complement activation, and intravascular coagulation.

C. Diagnosis

1. Clinical presentation

    a. Envenomation usually produces pain at the site within minutes, although it may be delayed.

    b. Occasionally, an erythematous or violaceous reaction surrounded by a ring of pallor ("halo," "target," or "bull's eye" lesion) may be seen at the bite site soon after envenomation.

    c. Necrosis with induration and eschar formation may develop several hours to 2 weeks after the bite.

    d. The eschar subsequently falls off, leaving an ulceration that may take months to heal. Many patients present at this stage and report having been bitten by "something."

    e. Systemic effects, although rare, may develop within hours after the bite and include fever, chills, headache, malaise, weakness, nausea, vomiting, arthralgia, myalgia, and rash.

        (1) These signs and symptoms may progress over 24 to 48 hours and usually resolve by 72 to 96 hours.

        (2) Laboratory findings may include anemia, thrombocytopenia, leukocytosis, and evidence of hemolysis and consumptive coagulopathy.

2. Evaluation

    a. There are no specific tests that can confirm or exclude envenomation. The diagnosis is based on the history and clinical findings.

    b. Routine laboratory studies include CBC, electrolytes, BUN, and creatinine. Patients with systemic symptoms should also have coagulation/disseminated intravascular coagulation (DIC) studies and haptoglobin/urinalysis for hemolysis.

3. Differential diagnosis

    a. Envenomation by many other spider species can produce a syndrome ("necrotic arachnadism") similar to that caused by the BRS.

    b. Other bites (most often arthropod or bug bites) and envenomations, infections (cellulitis, gonorrhea, herpes simplex, Lyme disease), and conditions (diabetes, emboli, foreign bodies, frostbite, vasculitis) and drugs (bromine, coumadin, heparin, ergot alkaloids) that can cause necrotic skin ulcers may be mistakenly diagnosed as BRS envenomation or necrotic arachnadism.

D. Management

1. Advanced life support measures should be provided as needed.

    a. Patients with systemic symptoms should be admitted.

    b. Those without systemic symptoms who present immediately after a bite should have wound checks as outpatients for 3 to 5 days following the bite.

2. Wound care is the same as for crotaline snakebites.

    a. Early surgical intervention (wide local excision) is not recommended.

    b. Dapsone, a leukocyte inhibitor, has been used to prevent ulceration without strong evidence of benefit.

3. The treatment of systemic arachnidism is mainly symptomatic and supportive.

    a. Corticosteroids (methylprednisolone or equivalent, 0.5 to 1 mg/kg IV every 6 hours) ameliorate hemolysis and are usually required for only 3 to 7 days.

> **b.** Alkalinization of the urine and aggressive hydration can protect against renal failure secondary to hemoglobinuria.
>
> **c.** Anemia and thrombocytopenia should be treated with packed red cells and platelets as needed. Whole blood and fresh-frozen plasma contain proteins that may react with venom components and contribute to red blood cell destruction and are not recommended.
>
> **d.** In severe coagulopathy, consult a hematologist regarding therapies such as antithrombin III or recombinant factor VIIa.

E. Complications

1. Wound healing may take several weeks to months. Revisions or cosmetic procedures may be considered if standard wound care fails.
2. Hemolysis may result in hemoglobinuria, renal failure, and shock or indirectly cause congestive heart failure, coma, convulsions, liver injury, and death as a result of anemic hypoxia.

V. SCORPION ENVENOMATION

A. Background

1. The bark scorpion (*Centruroides exilicauda*, formerly known as *C. sculpturatus*) is the only scorpion in the United States that produces systemic effects.
   a. Envenomation by other species causes only local effects.
   b. Scorpions grab the victim with pincers and repeatedly inject venom through the tail stinger.
2. *C. exilicauda* is usually about 5 cm in size, has a uniform tan, yellow, or brown color, and is found throughout the southwest (and northern Mexico), including Arizona, Texas, New Mexico, California, and Nevada.
3. Like spiders, scorpions may stow away and envenomations can happen elsewhere.
4. Several thousand scorpion envenomations occur in the United States each year. Severe reactions are mainly seen in children under age 10 years.

B. Pathophysiology

1. *C. exilicauda* venom contains neurotoxins that bind to sodium channels, resulting in activation of sympathetic, parasympathetic, and somatic motor neurons.
2. In contrast to some scorpions, it contains very little tissue necrotic factor.

C. Diagnosis

1. Clinical presentation
   a. Envenomation typically causes immediate local pain, which can usually be greatly exacerbated by tapping at the site of envenomation.
   b. Parasthesias develop within minutes to hours and may be generalized.
   c. Autonomic effects include tachycardia, excessive secretions, and, occasionally, vomiting and wheezing, salivation, and lacrimation.
   d. Somatic motor findings include roving eye movements, blurred vision, fasciculations (especially of the tongue), and poor control of pharyngeal and respiratory muscles.

    e. Stridor, hypoxia, aspiration, and respiratory arrest can occur in severe cases. Pancreatitis, rhabdomyolysis, and myocarditis have also been reported.

    f. Severity can be graded as follows:

        (1) Grade I: Local pain and/or paresthesias.

        (2) Grade II: Pain and/or paresthesias remote from the site of the sting.

        (3) Grade III: Either cranial nerve dysfunction (blurred vision, wandering eye movements, hypersalivation, tongue fasciculations, dysphagia, dysarthria, stridor) or somatic neuromuscular dysfunction (jerking of extremity[ies], restlessness).

        (4) Grade IV: Both cranial nerve and somatic neuromuscular dysfunction.

2. Evaluation

    a. There are no specific tests that can confirm or exclude envenomation. The diagnosis is based on the history and clinical findings.

    b. In severe cases, obtain CBC, electrolytes, BUN, creatinine, amylase and/or lipase, creatine kinase, and an electrocardiogram.

3. Differential diagnosis

    a. Severe involuntary shaking and jerking may be mistaken for seizures.

    b. Lack of a target skin lesion and continuous (as opposed to intermittent) writhing may help distinguish scorpion envenomation from that of the BWS.

    c. Respiratory symptoms are similar to those of intrinsic pulmonary conditions (i.e., asthma).

    d. Cholinergic and adrenergic symptoms are similar to those of intoxication by agents that have similar effects (e.g., organophosphate pesticides, sympathomimetics).

D. Management

1. Advanced life support measures should be provided as needed.

    a. Respiratory distress associated with hypersalivation has been treated with atropine, which may obviate the need endotracheal intubation.

    b. Patients with grade I or II envenomations should be observed for 3 to 4 hours after a sting for evidence of progression of symptoms. Those who do not manifest systemic symptoms can be discharged.

    c. Intensive care unit admission is recommended for patients with grade III or IV envenomations.

2. Wound care is the same as that for other envenomations.

3. Grade I or II envenomations are treated symptomatically.

    a. Application of ice to the sting often provides relief.

    b. Oral analgesics are effective in most cases, but parenteral analgesics may sometimes be needed.

    c. Steroids, epinephrine, calcium, and antihistamines have not been shown to be of benefit.

4. *C. sculpturatus* goat serum antivenom may be available for the treatment of grade III or IV envenomations in Arizona.

    a. It is administered IV but is no longer produced and stocks are diminishing.

    b. Signs and symptoms usually resolve within 30 to 90 minutes of administration.

    c. Although skin testing with antivenom is suggested, it is not completely reliable in predicting which patients will suffer allergic reactions. Those with a history of prolonged exposure to goats or goat's milk and those who have previously received goat serum antivenom are at increased risk for allergic reactions and should not be given antivenom.

    d. Up to 60% of patients treated with antivenom will go on to develop serum sickness.

  5. Grade III or IV envenomations can also be successfully treated with IV opiates and benzodiazepines and supportive care. Symptoms typically resolve in 4 to 20 hours.

E. Complications

  A. Secondary complications include respiratory failure and aspiration pneumonia.

  B. The time course and treatment of serum sickness in patients treated with *C. sculpturatus* antivenom is the same as that for those who receive crotaline antivenom.

Selected Readings
Crotaline Snake Envenomation

Dart RC, Seifert SA, Boyer LV, et al. A randomized multicenter trial of crotalinae polyvalent immune Fab (ovine) antivenom for the treatment for crotaline snakebite in the United States. *Arch Intern Med* 2001;161:2030–2036.
This article summarizes the efficacy and adverse effects of Fab antivenom therapy.

McKinney PE. Out-of-hospital and interhospital management of crotaline snakebite. *Ann Emerg Med* 2001;37(2):168–174.
A critical review of the treatment of crotaline envenomation, including first aid measures.

Ruha AM, Curry SC, Beuhler M, et al. Initial postmarketing experience with crotalidae polyvalent immune Fab for treatment of rattlesnake envenomation. *Ann Emerg Med* 2002;39(6):609–615.
This article summarizes the efficacy and adverse effects of Fab antivenom therapy.

Elipidae Envenomation

Kitchens CS, Van Mierop LHS. Envenomation by the Eastern coral snake (*Micrurus fulvius fulvius*). A study of 39 victims. *JAMA* 1987;258:1615–1618.
This is a review of the clinical manifestations and treatment of coral snake envenomation in the United States.

Black Widow Spider Envenomation

Clark RF, Wethern-Kestner S, Vance MV, et al. Clinical presentation and treatment of black widow spider envenomation: a review of 163 cases. *Ann Emerg Med* 1992;21(7):782–787.
Clark RF. The safety and efficacy of antivenin *Latrodectus mactans*. *J Toxicol Clin Toxicol* 2001;39(2):125–127.
These articles summarize the manifestations and management of black widow spider envenomation.

Brown Recluse Spider Envenomation

Wasserman G. Wound care of spider and snake envenomations. *Ann Emerg Med* 1988; 17:1331–1335.
This article reviews the options and controversies regarding local therapies for necrotic arachnidism.

Wright SW, Wrenn KD, Murray L, et al. Clinical presentation and outcome of brown recluse spider bite. *Ann Emerg Med* 1997;30(1):28–32.
This reference summarizes the authors' experience with 111 cases of suspected brown recluse spider envenomation.

Scorpion Envenomation

Bond GR. Antivenin administration for *Centruroides* scorpion sting: risks and benefits. *Ann Emerg Med* 1992;21:788–791.
This article summarizes and compares the use of antivenom with supportive care for the treatment of bark scorpion envenomation.

LoVecchio F, McBride C. Scorpion envenomation in young children in central Arizona. *J Toxicol Clin Toxicol* 2003;41:937–940.
This article describes the clinical findings and treatment of bark scorpion envenomation in children.

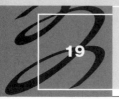

19 HEAVY METAL POISONING
Ivan E. Liang

I. LEAD

A. Background
1. Lead is found in elemental, inorganic, and organic forms and as a contaminant of other metals.
2. Lead-contaminated house dust is the major source of exposure for children.
3. Other common sources include lead curtain weights, fishing weights, bullets, and fragments from metal or machine shops.
4. Occupational exposure occurs in metal workers, renovators who clean or sandblast structures (aerosolization of lead), and those who produce lead-glazed pottery and glassware.
5. Traditional folk remedies may contain lead (e.g., azarcon, greta)
6. Lead poisoning is almost always the result of chronic ingestion or inhalation (fume, dust) exposure.
   a. Iron and calcium deficiency may promote intestinal lead absorption.
   b. Lead is poorly absorbed through intact skin, but cases of poisoning from cosmetics (e.g., eye shadow) have been reported.
   c. Poisoning may also result from the dissolution and absorption of lead from retained bullets (in spinal or synovial fluid).

B. Pathophysiology
1. Absorbed lead is principally carried in the red blood cells, where it is redistributed to soft tissue and bone, across the blood–brain barrier, and across the placenta.
2. Elimination occurs by urinary excretion and demonstrates a two-phase pattern with an initial half-life of months (reflecting soft tissue elimination) and a terminal one of years (reflecting bone elimination).
3. Lead adversely affects multiple organ systems through a variety of mechanisms, including dysregulation of calcium (and thus many major signal transduction pathways), inhibition of heme biosynthesis, binding to sulfhydryl and carboxyl ligands of macromolecules, and production of reactive radical species.
4. Children are more susceptible to the effects of lead than adults are.

C. Diagnosis
1. Clinical presentation
   a. With high-dose exposure, patients may present with encephalopathy (with coma and seizures), crampy abdominal pain (lead colic),

anemia, hepatitis, and peripheral motor neuropathy (typically extensor wrist drop).

b. Low-dose exposure causes more subtle and nonspecific symptoms such as headache, difficulty concentrating, fatigue, malaise, anorexia, constipation, myalgias, vomiting, neurobehavioral delay (in children), and paresthesias.

c. Hematologic abnormalities include normochromic or microcytic anemia, often with basophilic stippling of red blood cells.

d. Acute and chronic renal insufficiency (including a Fanconi-like syndrome), with consequent gout and hypertension, can occur.

e. Reproductive effects include abnormal sperm production, increased rates of miscarriage, and low birth weight.

2. Evaluation

a. Laboratory studies should include complete blood count (CBC), electrolytes, blood urea nitrogen (BUN), creatinine, and urinalysis.

b. A whole blood lead level (drawn and stored in lead-free containers) should be obtained for all patients suspected of lead poisoning.

(1) Baseline ("normal") levels are less than 5 mcg/dL.

(2) Biochemical toxicity is associated with levels of 5 to 10 mcg/dL.

(3) Subtle neurobehavioral effects can occur at levels of 10 to 20 μg/mL.

(4) Overt toxicity is seen with levels of 40 to 80 mcg/dL, although patients with such levels can be asymptomatic.

(5) Encephalopathy and peripheral neuropathy are associated with levels above 100 mcg/dL.

c. Serum free erythrocyte protoporphyrin (FEP) or zinc protoporphyrin (ZPP) may also be elevated (higher than 35 mcg/dL) as a result of impaired heme synthesis, but this does not occur until several weeks after exposure. Thus, an elevated whole blood level with a normal FEP suggests a recent exposure.

d. Because lead is radiopaque, abdominal x-rays may reveal ingested lead.

e. Urinary lead excretion (normal is less than 50 mcg/day) is also increased in lead poisoning.

f. Patients with altered mental status should have fundoscopy and a cranial CT scan performed to assess for signs of increased intracranial pressure (papilledema and cerebral edema).

3. Differential diagnosis

a. Toxicity is similar to that caused by other heavy metals. Peripheral neuropathy from lead tends to be motor, whereas that resulting from arsenic is predominantly sensory (pain paresthesias).

b. Other toxic and nontoxic causes of encephalopathy and abdominal pain must also be considered.

D. Management

1. Advanced life support measures should be instituted as necessary.

a. Seizures should be treated with benzodiazepines or barbiturates.

    b. Measures to reduce increased intracranial pressure may include elevation of the head, hyperventilation, restriction of fluids, corticosteroids, and mannitol.

2. Decontamination.

    a. Whole bowel irrigation (see Chapter 1) should be considered for any radiopaque source in the gastrointestinal (GI) tract.

    b. Surgical removal may be necessary for lead foreign bodies.

3. Chelation therapy

    a. Chelation decreases blood levels and increases urinary excretion, but protocols vary and controlled trials showing a beneficial effect are lacking.

    b. Calcium ethylenediaminetetraacetatel (EDTA) and dimercaprol (2,3-dimercapto-1-propanol, British anti-Lewisite, or BAL) are indicated for encephalopathy.

        (1) EDTA (30 to 50 mg/kg/day) is administered intramuscularly (two or three divided doses) rather than by continuous infusion in those with increased intracranial pressure, because intravenous (IV) EDTA must be diluted and given with a large volume of fluid.

        (2) Treatment with intramuscular BAL (3 to 5 mg/kg) 4 hours before EDTA may scavenge lead mobilized by EDTA and prevent deterioration as BAL (but not EDTA) crosses the blood–brain barrier. The dose is repeated every 4 hours.

        (3) Therapy is continued for 5 days and repeated after a 2-day holiday (to allow for lead redistribution) until symptoms improve and the lead level remains below 50 μg/dL.

    c. Symptomatic patients without encephalopathy and asymptomatic patients with high lead levels (>55 μg/dL in children and >100 μg/dL in adults) can be treated similarly, using low-end doses of EDTA and BAL and longer holidays.

    d. Oral dimercaptosuccinic acid (DMSA, succimer, or Chemet) can also be used for the treatment of patients without encephalopathy.

        (1) The manufacturer recommends 10 mg/kg every 8 hours for 5 days, followed by 10 mg/kg per dose every 12 hours for an additional 14 days.

        (2) Some clinicians prefer to interrupt dosing every 5 days as described for EDTA and BAL.

    e. D-penicillamine (5 mg/kg up to 500 mg every 6 hours), another oral chelator, is less effective but can be used in patients who cannot tolerate succimer.

    f. Blood lead levels should be monitored weekly during and after chelation therapy.

        (1) In symptomatic patients, therapy should be continued until the lead level drops below 20 μg/dL in children and 40 μg/dL in adults.

        (2) Reinstitution of therapy, depending on the rebound in lead level, may be necessary.

    g. Effective treatment must include measures to prevent further exposure. This is the only treatment necessary in asymptomatic patients with moderately elevated lead levels (up to 45 μg/dL in children and 80 μg/mL in adults).

E. Complications
   1. Neurotoxic effects and renal failure may slowly resolve or improve with time but can be permanent.
   2. Chelators have potentially serious side effects, and consultation with a Poison Center or toxicologist is advised before administration.

II. ARSENIC

A. Background
   1. Arsenic is found in rodenticides, insecticides, herbicides, paints, veterinary medicinals, and folk remedies and naturally in Earth's crust.
   2. It is also present in drinking water and seafood and is used in the production of glass, metals, computer chips, and other products.
   3. Arsenic trioxide is used as a cancer chemotherapy agent.
   4. Arsenic most commonly exists as inorganic trivalent (arsenite) and pentavalent (arsenate) salts and organometallic compounds.
      a. Pentavalent arsenic is less toxic than the trivalent form, although it may undergo biotransformation to trivalent arsenic.
      b. Seafood contains arsenobetaine, a methylated form of arsenic without known toxic effects.
   5. Arsine gas is formed when arsenic compounds interact with acids.
   6. Acute poisoning usually results from industrial accidents or suicidal or homicidal ingestion.

B. Pathophysiology
   1. Arsenic is a cellular toxin that acts in multiple ways to disrupt the enzymes responsible for oxidative phosphorylation.
   2. It is readily absorbed through the GI tract and through the lungs. Transdermal absorption is rare.
   3. Arsenic is eliminated primarily by renal excretion, which begins promptly after absorption and, depending on the amount of arsenic ingested, may remain elevated for 1 to 2 months.

C. Diagnosis
   1. Clinical presentation
      a. Arsenic has a metallic taste and garlicky odor and is extremely irritating to the GI tract. Significant ingestions lead to abdominal pain, nausea, and vomiting and may progress to hemorrhagic gastroenteritis.
      b. Cardiovascular effects include hypotension, cardiogenic shock, and ventricular tachyarrhythmias.
         (1) Electrocardiographic (ECG) changes associated with arsenic poisoning include ST and T wave changes, which may mimic ischemia or hyperkalemia, and QTc prolongation with torsades de pointes.
         (2) These abnormalities occur 4 to 30 hours postingestion and can persist for up to 8 weeks.
      c. Both noncardiogenic and cardiogenic pulmonary edema may occur.
      d. Pancytopenia can occur, achieving a nadir at 1 to 2 weeks postexposure, with recovery at 2 to 3 weeks after the nadir.

e. Arsine gas inhalation results in rapid and severe Coombs' negative hemolytic anemia.

f. Delirium, convulsions, encephalopathy, and coma may be seen with acute poisoning.

g. Polyneuropathy, traditionally described as an axonal-loss sensorimotor polyneuropathy (low amplitude/unelicitable sensory and motor conduction responses, often with preserved motor conduction velocities), can occur after acute or chronic exposure.

   (1) Symptoms range from mild "stocking glove" paresthesias to extreme pain provoked by minor sensory stimuli.

   (2) Ascending weakness and paralysis may occasionally occur.

h. Renal dysfunction may result from hypovolemia, shock, direct toxicity, or hemoglobinuria from hemolysis resulting from arsine.

i. Dermal effects include patchy hyperpigmentation ("raindrops on a dusty road"), hyperkeratosis (palms and feet), and, rarely, skin cancer. The lesions usually appear 1 to 6 weeks after exposure. Brittle nails with transverse white bands known Reynolds–Aldrich–Mees lines as well as patchy alopecia may also develop.

2. Evaluation

a. Symptomatic patients should have CBC, electrolytes, BUN, creatinine, liver function studies, coagulation times, creatine phosphokinase, urinalysis, arterial blood gas, ECG, and chest x-ray.

b. Because arsenic is radiopaque, acute intentional ingestions should be assessed by abdominal x-ray.

c. Whole blood and urinary arsenic levels should also be obtained.

   (1) Blood arsenic levels are highly variable. Toxicity can occur with normal values (less than 5 mcg/L).

   (2) Elevated urinary arsenic in a single ("spot") urine sample (normal less than 30 mcg/L) or a 24-hour urinary collection (normal less than 50 mcg/L) supports the diagnosis.

   i. With acute poisoning, levels are typically greater than 1,000 mcg/L.

   ii. With chronic exposure, levels are typically lower.

   iii. Levels typically remain elevated for weeks.

   iv. Elevated levels resulting from nontoxic arsenobetaine can result from the recent (several days) ingestion of seafood.

   v. Identification (speciation) of the type of arsenic present may be sometimes necessary.

3. Differential diagnosis

a. Arsenic poisoning should be considered in patients with unexplained hemorrhagic gastroenteritis and multisystem organ failure.

b. Other toxins (salicylates, iron, mercury, toxalbumins) and nontoxic conditions (sepsis) should be considered in the differential diagnosis.

D. Management

1. Advanced life support measures should be instituted as necessary.

a. Patients with central nervous system (CNS) depression or unstable vitals signs may require endotracheal intubation.

b. Aggressive cardiovascular support with IV fluids, blood products, pressors, and antiarrhythmics (see Chapter 4) may also be necessary.

2. Decontamination

a. Gastric lavage (see Chapter 1) is recommended for patients with recent, acute, intentional ingestion, particularly if radiopaque material is visible on abdominal x-ray.

b. Surgical removal (gastrotomy) should be considered if radiopaque material remains despite gastric lavage.

3. Chelation therapy

a. BAL, the traditional arsenic chelating agent, is most effective when administered promptly (i.e., within minutes to hours) after acute arsenic exposure.

(1) In patients with acute symptomatic intoxication, treatment should not be delayed while waiting for laboratory confirmation.

(2) Dosing is the same as that described for lead.

b. Unithiol (2,3-dimercaptopropanesullonic acid, or DMPS), a water-soluble analog of BAL that can be administered IV (3 to 5 mg/kg over 20 minutes every 4 hours) can be given instead of BAL, but this formulation may be difficult to obtain.

c. If the patient is stable and can tolerate oral fluids, DMSA (or d-penicillamine) should be administered in the same dosing regimen as described for lead.

d. Therapeutic end points of chelation therapy are poorly defined. Patients with acute exposure should be treated until symptoms resolve and urinary arsenic levels approach normal.

4. Hemodialysis may be necessary in patients with renal insufficiency.

5. Prompt exchange transfusion with whole blood may significantly aid hemolysis and renal failure following arsine gas exposure.

E. Complications

1. Neurotoxic effects may be delayed in onset, particularly following chronic exposure, and may not respond to chelation therapy.

2. Multisystem organ failure may occur.

III. MERCURY

A. Background

1. Mercury is encountered in elemental as well as inorganic (salt) and organic forms.

2. It is used in laboratory and industrial settings and in older thermometers, dental amalgam, and herbicide, fungicide, and antiseptic formulations.

3. Methylmercury is bioaccumulated in carnivorous fish (e.g., salmon, swordfish, tuna).

B. Pathophysiology

1. Mercury reacts with sulfhydryl moieties of proteins, leading to nonspecific inhibition of enzyme systems and pathologic alteration of cellular membranes.

2. Poisoning can result from acute or chronic exposure.

3. Elemental mercury is a liquid at room temperature and is easily volatilized.

  a. It is not absorbed from the gut, but inhalation can result in pulmonary irritation as well as systemic toxicity.

  b. Injection, which can cause similar toxicity, has also been reported.

  c. Absorption from silver-mercury amalgam tooth fillings is negligible.

4. Inorganic and organic mercury are absorbed following ingestion.

  a. Mercury salts can cause skin, mucous membrane, and GI tract irritation as well as systemic effects.

  b. Methylmercury is particularly toxic to the developing fetus and to infants.

C. Diagnosis

1. Clinical toxicity

  a. Elemental mercury

  (1) Toxicity does not result from ingestion unless mercury escapes from the gut (e.g., through a perforation) or remains there for prolonged periods (e.g., becomes trapped in the appendix or diverticula).

  (2) In the gut and tissues, it is slowly converted to organic mercury.

  (3) Acute high-dose inhalation of mercury vapor may result in chemical pneumonitis, noncardiogenic pulmonary edema, and gingivostomatitis.

  (4) Chronic low-dose inhalation may result in acrodynia ("pink disease") characterized by redness of the palms and soles, edema of the hands and feet, rashes, diaphoresis, tachycardia, hypertension, photophobia, irritability, emotional instability, memory loss, insomnia, and anorexia.

  (5) Nausea, vomiting, diarrhea, renal failure, pneumonitis, constriction of visual fields, discoloration of the lens capsule, dermatitis, and tremor can also occur.

  b. Inorganic mercury

  (1) Acute ingestion of large doses typically causes abrupt onset of hemorrhagic gastroenteritis, subsequent hypovolemic shock, and oliguric renal failure from acute tubular necrosis.

  (2) Chronic ingestion of low doses may result in acrodynia (see earlier).

  c. Organic mercury

  (1) Toxicity usually results from chronic ingestion and is insidious in onset.

  (2) Neurologic effects include paresthesias, confusion, hallucinosis, irritability, sleep disturbances, ataxia, memory loss, slurred speech, auditory defects, narrowing of visual fields, emotional instability, and inability to concentrate.

  (3) Ethylmercury can also cause nonspecific GI complaints.

  (4) Perinatal exposure to methylmercury can result in mental retardation and a cerebral palsy–like syndrome.

2. Evaluation

  a. Laboratory studies in patients with suspected mercury poisoning should include CBC, electrolytes, BUN, creatinine, and urinalysis.

b. Mercury is radiopaque, and radiographic studies may confirm ingestion or injection. The absence of radiographic visualization does not
exclude exposure, however.

c. Whole blood and urinary mercury concentrations are used to confirm exposure.

   (1) Normal whole blood, "spot" urine, and 24-hour urine mercury
   concentrations are usually less than 2 μg/dL, 10 μg/L, and 50 μg/
   24 hours, respectively. Higher levels can be seen in those with
   occupational exposure and after acute or chronic carnivorous fish
   consumption.

   (2) With acute poisoning, the whole blood level is usually greater
   than 50 μg/dL and urinary levels range from hundreds to thou-
   sands.

   (3) With chronic exposure, urine mercury concentrations between
   30 and 50 μg/L may be associated with subclinical neuropsychiatric effects, levels of 50 to 100 μg/L may be associated with
   subclinical tremor, levels greater than 100 μg/L may be associated with overt neuropsychiatric disturbances, and those greater
   than 200 μg/L are usually associated with true tremors.

   (4) Chronic toxicity is usually associated with blood levels greater
   than 20 μg/dL.

3. Differential diagnosis

   a. The differential diagnosis is the same as for arsenic poisoning.

   b. Subtle neurologic and neuropsychiatric complaints should prompt
   specific questioning regarding possible heavy metal exposure.

D. Management

1. Supportive care, decontamination, and complications are similar to
those described for arsenic.

   a. Patients who have visible elemental mercury in the gut or tissue on
   radiographs should initially have follow-up radiographs and/or mercury levels checked every few months.

   b. If mercury levels increase or mercury remains visible in the gut, surgical removal can be performed.

2. Chelation therapy

   a. BAL, DMSA, DMPS, and d-penicillamine are all effective in enhancing mercury excretion.

   b. Doses and treatment considerations are the same as for arsenic.

3. Oral N-acetylcysteine (see Chapter 2), a sulfhydryl donor, may be of
benefit for organic and inorganic mercury exposures.

Selected Readings
Lead

Canfield RL, Gendle MH, Cory-Slechta DA. Impaired neuropsychological functioning
in lead-exposed children. *Dev Neuropsychol* 2004;26(1):513–540.
   *This study shows that low blood lead levels can have adverse effects on intellectual
   function in children.*

Graziano JH. Role of 2,3-dimercaptosuccinic acid in the treatment of heavy metal poisoning. *Med Toxicol* 1986;1:155–162.
   This paper reviews the pharmacology and use of DMSA in heavy metal poisoning.

Lin JL, Ho HH, Yu CC. Chelation therapy for patients with elevated body lead burden and progressive renal insufficiency. A randomized, controlled trial. *Ann Intern Med* 1999;130(1):7–13.
This study suggests that chelation therapy slows the progression of renal insufficiency in adults with mildly elevated lead levels.

Arsenic

Beckman KJ, Bauman JL, Pimental PA, et al. Arsenic-induced torsade de pointes. *Crit Care Med* 1991;19:290–292.
Case report and discussion of the electrophysiologic toxicity of arsenic.

Kyle RA, Pease GL. Hematologic aspects of arsenic intoxication. *N Engl J Med* 1965;273:18–23.
This article reviews the hemotologic toxicity of arsenic.

Stephanopoulos DE, Willman DA, Shevlin D, Pinter L, Gummin DD. Treatment and toxicokinetics of acute pediatric arsenic ingestion: danger of arsenic insecticides in children. *Pediatr Crit Care Med* 2002 Jan;3:74–80.
Case report and discussion of supportive care and chelation therapy in severe arsenic poisoning.

Mercury

Counter SA, Buchanan LH. Mercury exposure in children: a review. *Toxicol Appl Pharmacol* 2004 Jul 15;198(2):209–230.
Review of the sources, toxicity, and treatment of acute and chronic mercury exposure in children.

Dodes JE. The amalgam controversy. An evidence-based analysis. *J Am Dent Assoc* 2001;132:348–356.
This critical review of the literature pertaining to silver–mercury dental amalgams concluded that they are safe and effective.

McFee RB, Caraccio TR. Intravenous mercury injection and ingestion: clinical manifestations and management. *J Toxicol Clin Toxicol* 2001;39:733–738.
Discusses the toxicity and treatment of mercury injection and ingestion.

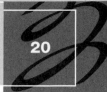

I. BACKGROUND

A. Hydrofluoric acid is a weak acid ($pK_a = 3.8$) that is available in concentrations ranging from less than 10% to more than 99% (anhydrous). Hydrofluoric acid produces fumes at concentrations greater than 48%.

   1. Dilute solutions are used as household rust removers.

   2. Concentrated solutions are used for glass etching, in semiconductor manufacturing, as a brick cleaner, and in the production of high-octane fuels.

B. Hydrofluoric acid can cause systemic fluoride poisoning as well as local corrosive injury.

C. Death has occurred in adults with body surface area (BSA) burns of less than 2.5% from concentrated hydrofluoric acid and ingestions of more than 3 ounces of dilute hydrofluoric acid.

D. Air concentrations of 200 ppm result in severe distress, and concentrations of 12,000 ppm are likely to be rapidly fatal.

E. Ammonium fluoride and ammonium bifluoride have similar uses and toxicity.

II. PATHOPHYSIOLOGY

A. Liberated protons cause liquefactive necrosis of skin, gastric mucosa, and respiratory tract and contribute to systemic acidosis.

B. The highly electronegative fluoride ion (F^-) binds tissue Ca^{2+} and Mg^{2+}, forming insoluble salts and resulting in pain, hypocalcemia, and hypomagnesemia.

C. F^- disrupts the Na^+/K^+-ATPase pump and Ca^{2+}-dependent K^+ channels, leading to hyperkalemia.

D. F^- also interferes with multiple enzyme functions, resulting in cell death.

III. DIAGNOSIS

A. Clinical Presentation

   1. Systemic toxicity

      a. May develop following dermal exposure and inhalation as well as ingestion.

      b. Massive exposures to concentrated hydrofluoric acid are associated with syncope and rapid death.

   c. Systemic effects may be delayed up to 4 hours after ingestion of dilute solutions or dermal exposures to concentrated hydrofluoric acid.

   d. Fatalities result from severe hypocalcemia, hypomagnesemia, and hyperkalemia, as well as acute pulmonary injury.

   e. Carpopedal spasm, positive Chvostek and Trousseau signs, hyperreflexia, and tetany may result from hypocalcemia.

   f. Coma, seizures, shock, ventricular tachycardia, ventricular fibrillation, and pulseless electrical activity (PEA) can occur.

2. Dermal exposure

   a. Signs and symptoms may be delayed up to 24 hours following exposure to dilute (less than 20%) hydrofluoric acid. Patients present with pain out of proportion to examination, which may reveal erythema, edema, or whitish-blue discoloration.

   b. Immediate pain develops with exposure to concentrations higher than 49%, and findings include blistering, black eschar, or areas of subcutaneous liquefactive necrosis appearing as firm white areas.

3. Ingestion

   a. Unintentional ingestion of small amounts of dilute hydrofluoric acid may not cause significant gastrointestinal (GI) distress, whereas intentional ingestions of larger volumes typically cause abdominal pain and vomiting. Despite the potential absence of GI symptoms with dilute ingestions, serious systemic poisoning may occur within 1 to 4 hours.

   b. Concentrated solutions produce immediate caustic injury to oral, esophageal, and gastric mucosa and are likely to result in significant systemic poisoning.

4. Ocular exposure

   a. Can occur with splashes of hydrofluoric acid as well as fumes.

   b. Dilute exposures may induce pain, tearing, conjunctival injection, and corneal erosions.

   c. Concentrated exposures can result in severe corneal injury with opacification, ulceration, perforation, and anterior chamber involvement.

5. Inhalation

   a. Exposure to hydrofluoric acid fumes typically produces immediate airway irritation with throat pain, coughing, choking, and bronchospasm.

   b. Pulmonary edema may follow but can be delayed by several hours.

B. Evaluation

1. Symptomatic patients with ingesting inhalation exposure and dermal burns from concentrated hydrofluoric acid exceeding 1% BSA are at risk for systemic toxicity and require ancillary testing.

   a. Initiate cardiac monitoring and obtain an electrocardiogram (ECG) to assess for hypocalcemia (prolonged QT interval) and hyperkalemia (QRS widening and peaked T waves).

   b. Measure serum calcium (ionized is preferred), magnesium, and potassium as well as other serum electrolytes, blood urea nitrogen (BUN), creatinine, and glucose.

   c. In patients with persistent symptoms or initial laboratory abnormalities, these evaluations should be repeated every 30 to 60 minutes for 4 to 6 hours or until normalization occurs.

2. Dermal burns from dilute hydrofluoric acid covering less than 5% BSA do not require such testing.

3. Chest radiographs are indicated for any respiratory symptoms to assess for pulmonary edema.

4. Serum fluoride concentrations are not readily available nor helpful in management.

IV. TREATMENT

A. Advanced Life Support Measures should be instituted as necessary.

1. Patients at risk for systemic toxicity (see earlier) should receive empiric intravenous (IV) calcium added to initial IV fluids, pending laboratory results. Give 20 mL of 10% calcium gluconate in 1 L of crystalloid (0.2 mL/kg in 10 mL/kg of crystalloid in children) over 1 hour.

2. Those with clinical or laboratory evidence of hypocalcemia should receive bolus therapy with 10% calcium gluconate (0.2 mL/kg). In stable patients, the dose should be given over 5 to 10 minutes. In unstable patients, it should be given rapid push. The dose should be repeated until symptoms resolve or the serum calcium level is normalized.

3. Ten percent calcium chloride may also be used, preferably via central vein catheter because it is more irritating to veins (and tissue, if extravasated). It contains about three times more calcium than the gluconate salt (13.6 mEq/10 mL versus 4.6 mEq/10 mL for calcium gluconate) so the equivalent dose is 0.07 mL/kg. The chloride salt may be preferable for severe poisoning, which may require massive amounts of calcium (several hundred milliequivalents in 24 hours).

4. Magnesium replacement may be given as 2 g of the sulfate salt in 100 cc of 0.9% NaCl over 10 minutes (25 to 50 mg/kg in 10 mg/mL of saline or D5W for children). Because serum Mg^{2+} may not accurately reflect available Mg^{2+}, loss of knee-jerk reflex can be used to mark adequate therapy.

5. In addition to calcium, hyperkalemia should be treated with insulin, glucose, and bicarbonate according to standard protocols.

B. Decontamination

1. Contaminated clothing should be removed, and patients should have the affected area thoroughly irrigated with water for at least 20 minutes.

2. One liter of saline irrigation is recommended for ocular exposures.

3. Optimal GI decontamination is unknown. Small amounts of water may be given for accidental ingestions. Another option of unproved benefit is to administer oral calcium or magnesium (10% calcium gluconate, magnesium or calcium antacids), which may bind F^- and prevent absorption.

C. Dermal Exposures

1. Calcium salts are delivered through a variety of techniques with the goals of binding fluoride, providing pain relief, and preventing further tissue destruction.

a. First-line therapy is topical application of 2.5% to 10% calcium gluconate gel (prepared by crushing tablets and mixing with K-Y Jelly if a commercial preparation is unavailable). Cover the burn with gel and apply an occlusive dressing. For hand burns, a surgical glove filled with gel can be used. If pain is relieved, continue to apply every 4 hours for 24 hours. Lack of pain relief after 1 hour indicates the need for alternative therapy.

b. Local injection of 5% calcium gluconate (0.5 mL/cm^2 of tissue using a 27- or 30-gauge needle) may provide relief in areas where injected fluid volume will not pose a risk of tissue damage. Fingers and toes should be avoided for this reason.

c. IV regional perfusion using the Bier block technique can provide adequate calcium delivery to tissues where local injection is not possible (fingers, toes, nail beds) or is impractical (large surface area extremity burns). Obtain IV access in the affected extremity. Elevate the extremity and exsanguinate using an Esmarch bandage (or occlude the brachial/femoral artery while the limb is elevated to prevent further flow and allow venous drainage), followed by inflation of a tourniquet to 50 mmHg above the patient's systolic blood pressure to prevent reperfusion. Infuse 10 to 15 mL of calcium gluconate in 50 mL D5W or normal saline (proportionately less in children) and slowly release the tourniquet 20 to 30 minutes later. Constant monitoring is necessary during the procedure to ensure that cuff pressure is stable. Significant pain may develop from the tourniquet as well as the calcium infusion. Procedural sedation may be necessary.

d. Intraarterial calcium is potentially the most effective technique for digit burns, particularly when nail beds are involved. After ensuring adequate collateral flow to the hand (Allen test), insert a radial arterial line and verify placement by monitoring the arterial waveform. Infuse 10 mL of calcium gluconate in 50 mL D5W or normal saline (proportionately less in children) over 4 hours. Ulnar-sided injuries can be treated in this way if good collateral flow exists. Patients typically require several 4-hour infusions for lasting pain relief. If pain is not relieved after four infusions, the technique is unlikely to provide further benefit. Intensive care unit procedures are necessary to safely monitor the arterial line.

2. Adequate analgesia may require adjunctive opioids or regional anesthesia such as digital blocks.

D. Ingestion

1. Patients with GI symptoms or mucosal burns require GI consultation for endoscopy (see Chapter 15).

2. Patients who remain or become asymptomatic and have a normal serum calcium level 4 to 6 hours after exposure may be discharged or medically cleared for psychiatric evaluation.

E. Ocular Exposure

1. Ophthalmology consultation is indicated for all exposures.

2. There is no evidence to support the use of topical calcium salts in the eye.

F. Inhalation
   1. Respiratory injuries are treated with usual symptomatic and supportive measures.
   2. Nebulized calcium gluconate (2.5%; 1.5 mL of 10% calcium gluconate + 4.5 mL 0.9% NaCl) may provide some benefit and has no known adverse effects.

V. COMPLICATIONS

   A. Permanent disfigurement and disability, particularly of the digits, may result from severe dermal burns.
   B. Ocular burns can cause permanent vision impairment or complete vision loss.

Selected Readings

Graudins A, Burns MJ, Aaron CK. Regional intravenous infusion of calcium gluconate for hydrofluoric acid burns of the upper extremity. *Ann Emerg Med* 1997;30: 604–607.
   Case series that discusses the efficacy of regional IV calcium therapy for hydrofluoric acid dermal burns.

Vance MV, Curry SC, Kunkel DB, et al. Digital hydrofluoric acid burns: treatment with intraarterial calcium infusion. *Ann Emerg Med* 1986;15(8):890–896.
   Case series describing the technique and efficacy of intraarterial calcium infusion for fingertip injuries from hydrofluoric acid.

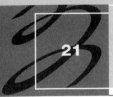

21 HYDROCARBONS
D. Eric Brush

I. BACKGROUND

A. Hydrocarbons commonly involved in poisoning include a variety of aliphatic, halogenated, and aromatic compounds and terpenes (Table 21-1).

    1. Aliphatic hydrocarbons are straight-chain compounds obtained from petroleum distillation and used as adhesives, solvents, and fuels.

    2. Halogenated hydrocarbons are aliphatic or aromatic derivatives containing one or more atoms of chlorine, bromine, fluorine, or iodine and used as solvents and refrigerants (e.g., Freon).

    3. Aromatic hydrocarbons contain one or more benzene rings and are common constituents of glues and paints.

    4. Terpenes are plant-derived cyclic hydrocarbons formed by joining isoprene (C_5H_8) units and are found in solvents and household cleaners.

B. Poisoning may result from ingestion, inhalation, or dermal or ocular exposure.

II. PATHOPHYSIOLOGY

A. Pulmonary Toxicity

    1. Aspiration usually occurs during ingestion or subsequent vomiting.

    2. Inhalation is less likely to cause pulmonary injury, but it can occur with high concentrations or prolonged exposure.

    3. Inhibition of surfactant leads to alveolar collapse and ventilation perfusion mismatch. Chemical pneumonitis results from direct capillary damage.

    4. Agents with a low viscosity and low surface tension spread easily to distal airways and cause pneumonitis, whereas highly viscous agents with high surface tension cause more localized (lipoid) pneumonia.

B. Central Nervous System Toxicity

    1. Hydrocarbons are readily absorbed following inhalation but poorly absorbed by other routes.

    2. They are highly lipophilic, rapidly enter the brain, and cause central nervous system (CNS) excitation followed by depression after systemic absorption.

C. Cardiac Toxicity. Myocardial sensitization to catecholamines can occur after exposure to halogenated and aromatic hydrocarbons, leading to ventricular irritability and dysrhythmias.

TABLE 21-1	Hydrocarbons

Aliphatic	Aromatic
N-hexane*	Benzene
N-butane*	Toluene*
Isobutane*	Xylene
Propane*	Diphenyl
Gasoline	Phenol
Charcoal lighter fluid	Styrene
Mineral spirits	**Terpenes**
Kerosene	Terpentine
Fuel oil	Pine oil
Naphtha	Camphor
Halogenated	
Carbon tetrachloride	
Chloroform	
Freon 12 (dichlorofluoromethane)	
Freon 11 (trichlorofluoromethane)	
Tetrachloroethylene (TCE)	
Trichloroethane (TCA)	

*Common volatile substance of abuse (VSA)

D. Dermal, Gastrointestinal, and Ocular Toxicity

1. Hydrocarbons have mild corrosive effects.

2. Metabolism of ingested or inhaled carbon tetrachloride via CYP450 enzymes leads to free-radical formation and subsequent hepatic necrosis.

III. DIAGNOSIS

A. Clinical Presentation

1. Pulmonary aspiration of even small amounts of hydrocarbons can lead to severe respiratory symptoms within 30 minutes. Peak effects occur within 24 to 48 hours and tend to resolve after 5 to 7 days.

   a. Symptoms include coughing, choking, vomiting, and dyspnea.

   b. Tachypnea, respiratory distress, rales or wheezing, fever, leukocytosis, and hypoxia are common findings.

   c. Pulmonary edema, chemical pneumonitis, and respiratory failure can occur in severe cases.

2. Inhalation of a volatile substance of abuse (VSA; Table 21-1) leads to rapid CNS effects including sedation, euphoria, dizziness, confusion, drowsiness, and, rarely, coma or seizure.

   a. Large ingestions or severe aspiration lead to similar CNS effects.

   b. Inhalation of halogenated hydrocarbons, benzene, and, less commonly, gasoline and toluene are associated with cardiac dysrhythmias. Ventricular fibrillation is the cause of "sudden sniffing death syndrome."

   c. Myocardial depression can be also seen.

    d. Chronic inhalational abuse may cause perioral frost, dermatitis, and pigmentation.

    e. Because of flammability, accidental burns may occur in careless recreational abusers.

  4. Gastrointestinal effects after ingestion include oropharyngeal irritation, nausea, vomiting, and abdominal pain.

  5. Hepatotoxicity from carbon tetrachloride becomes clinically evident between 2 to 4 days after acute exposure; however, it is more commonly seen with chronic exposures. Other hepatotoxic hydrocarbons include benzene, trichloroethylene, and pentane.

  6. Chronic inhalation of toluene can cause type IV renal tubular acidosis (bicarbonate wasting) with hypokalemia and rhabdomyolysis. Patients present with profound weakness.

  7. Hepatic metabolism of methylene chloride to carbon monoxide can cause elevated carboxyhemoglobin fractions (up to 50%), leading to cellular asphyxia (see Chapter 34).

  8. Dermal and ocular irritation occur after acute or chronic exposure.

B. Evaluation

  1. Oxygen saturation or arterial blood gas analysis and a chest radiograph should be obtained in all patients with respiratory symptoms or findings and when aspiration is suspected. These tests should be done immediately if respiratory symptoms are present or at 6 hours after exposure in asymptomatic patients to allow time for x-ray findings to develop. Findings may include focal atalectasis, basilar infiltrates, or pulmonary edema.

  2. Patients with altered mental status, respiratory distress, and hypoxia should also have cardiac monitoring.

  3. With ingestion, an abdominal radiograph may reveal two fluid levels in the stomach (double bubble sign) because these compounds are not water soluble and generally have a higher density than water. Halogenated hydrocarbons are radiopaque and may be seen in the GI tract.

  4. Patients with ocular exposures should have fluorescein staining and a slit lamp examination.

  5. Depending on the exposure and the nature of toxicity, a complete blood count (CBC), serum electrolytes, blood urea nitrogen (BUN), creatinine, glucose, hepatic profile, creatine phosphokinase (CPK) and cardiac markers, carboxyhemoglobin fraction, and urinalysis may be indicated.

  6. Hippuric acid crystals in the urine may be seen with toluene exposure.

IV. TREATMENT

  A. Advanced life support measures should be instituted as necessary.

  B. All patients with altered mental status, respiratory symptoms, or hypoxia should be given supplemental oxygen.

    1. Early intubation is indicated for significant respiratory distress.

    2. Mechanical ventilatory support is indicated when appropriate.

    3. Steroids have no proved benefit in the treatment of hydrocarbon aspiration.

4. Antibiotics are not routinely indicated. Their use should ideally be guided by cultures of sputum or bronchial lavage.

5. Asymptomatic patients who are suspected of aspirating hydrocarbons may be safely discharged if the chest radiograph is normal 6 hours after exposure.

C. Ventricular dysrhythmias should be treated with β-blockers, lidocaine, and benzodiazepines. Epinephrine may exacerbate myocardial irritability and should be avoided.

D. N-acetylcysteine (see Chapter 2) may be useful for the treatment of hepatotoxicity from carbon tetrachloride.

E. Activated charcoal is of limited use in preventing the absorption of hydrocarbons and is not recommended. Emesis is contraindicated because of the risk of aspiration. Gastric aspiration with a small-caliber nasogastric (NG) tube may be useful for large-volume ingestions (>30 mL) or for inherently toxic hydrocarbons described by the pneumonic CHAMP (camphor, halogenated, aromatic, metal containing, or pesticides in a hydrocarbon vehicle).

F. Saturated clothing should be immediately removed and the patient's skin washed with soap and water to limit dermal absorption.

G. The initial treatment of ocular exposures is irrigation (see Chapter 1).

V. COMPLICATIONS

A. Complications of aspiration include bacterial infection, pleural effusion, pneumatoceles, pneumothorax, and persistent respiratory dysfunction.

B. Chronic inhalation can lead to leukoencephalopathy characterized by cerebellar ataxia and encephalopathy or dementia.

C. Chronic inhalation, particularly of *n*-hexane, can also cause peripheral neuropathy.

D. Chronic exposure to benzene may cause bone marrow suppression and aplastic anemia and is linked to acute myelogenous leukemia.

Selected Reading

Anas N, Namasonthi V, Ginsburg CM. Criteria for hospitalizing children who have ingested products containing hydrocarbon. *JAMA* 1981;246:840–843.
This study observed patients who presented and remained asymptomatic after 6 to 8 hours of observation and who did not develop subsequent manifestations.

22

IRON

D. Eric Brush

I. BACKGROUND

  A. Iron is the leading cause of accidental poisoning death from pharmaceutical agents among young children.
   1. The amount of iron ion ingested correlates with toxicity.
   2. Iron salts vary in their iron ion content (Table 22-1).
   3. Ingestions of more than 20 mg/kg of ionized iron may produce significant gastrointestinal (GI) distress.
   4. Doses of 40 to 60 mg/kg or higher are potentially fatal.
  B. Multivitamin preparations contain relatively small amounts of iron salts and have not been associated with significant poisoning.
  C. Although iron carbonyl is almost pure iron, it consists of uncharged powdered elemental iron, which is insoluble and poorly absorbed (only after ionization by gastric acid) and has not resulted in significant toxicity.

II. PATHOPHYSIOLOGY

  A. Approximately 10% of ingested ferrous (Fe^{2+}) iron is absorbed (in the proximal small bowel). It is subsequently converted to the ferric (Fe^{3+}) state and joins with ferritin to form complexes in the intestinal mucosa. Transport to other tissues occurs through transfer and binding to serum transferrin. Normal serum iron concentrations range from 50 to 150 µg/dL.
  B. After overdose, transferrin becomes saturated and excess iron joins to form complexes with other plasma proteins or exists as free ferric ion. Peak serum iron concentrations typically occur within 4 to 6 hours, although delays are seen with sustained-release preparations.
  C. Free iron ferric ion disrupts oxidative phosphorylation and catalyzes the formation of oxygen free radicals, leading to lipid peroxidation and cell death. It also produces venodilation, increases capillary permeability, causes a shift to anaerobic metabolism through mitochondrial dysfunction, and generates hydrogen ions with hydration: $Fe^{3+} + 3H_2O \rightarrow Fe(OH)_3 + 3H^+$.
   1. GI symptoms result from damage to intestinal mucosal cells, similar to that resulting from corrosive injury.
   2. Shock results from GI fluid losses, volume redistribution ("third spacing"), vasodilation, and myocardial dysfunction.
   3. Hepatic necrosis results from injury resulting from free radical formation.

TABLE 22-1	Iron Preparations
Compound	**Percent iron**
Ferrous gluconate	12
Ferrous lactate	19
Ferrous sulfate	20
Ferrous chloride	28
Ferrous fumarate	33

4. Initial coagulopathy results from direct inhibition of coagulation factors by iron, whereas hepatic failure is responsible for later abnormalities in coagulation.

III. DIAGNOSIS

A. Clinical Toxicity

1. Iron poisoning is primarily a clinical diagnosis. It is commonly divided into five stages; however, stages do not always occur at predictable intervals following overdose, and they may be absent or overlap.

a. Stage 1: *GI symptoms* develop within hours of overdose and may include nausea, vomiting, hematemesis, diarrhea, and hematochezia.

b. Stage 2: In the *"quiescent phase,"* resolution of GI symptoms may occur. This phase may persist up to 24 hours following ingestion. Laboratory monitoring may reveal progressive metabolic acidosis.

c. Stage 3: *Shock* occurs and progressive cardiovascular decompensation may ensue.

d. Stage 4: *Hepatotoxicity* may occur at any time within the first 48 hours following overdose.

e. Stage 5: *Gastrointestinal scarring and stricture formation* may result in gastric outlet or small bowel obstruction 2 to 4 weeks after overdose.

2. Peak serum iron concentrations tend to correlate with clinical toxicity (Table 22-2).

TABLE 22-2	Interpretation of Serum Iron Concentration
Serum concentration (μg/dL)	**Expected toxicity**
<300	Often asymptomatic
300–500	Significant GI, moderate systemic
500–1,000	Severe GI, shock
>1,000	Shock and possible death
10,000	Death almost universal

3. Findings that correlate with a serum iron concentration higher than 300 to 500 µg/dL, in order of decreasing sensitivity, include coma or central nervous system (CNS) depression, increased anion gap (greater than 15), metabolic acidosis, radiopacities indicative of iron tablets on abdominal radiograph, leukocytosis (white blood count above 15,000/mm^3), hyperglycemia (serum glucose higher than 150 mg/dL), and protracted or persistent vomiting or diarrhea.

   a. Except for coma, individual findings have low positive predictive values, but taken collectively they have a high negative predictive one.

   b. A serum iron level exceeding the total iron binding capacity (TIBC) is not a useful parameter for iron overdose.

4. The fetus may be relatively protected from overdose during pregnancy because transplacental iron delivery requires active transport, and this pathway is saturated in overdose. Fetal health depends on maternal condition.

B. Evaluation

1. Obtain complete blood count (CBC), serum electrolytes, glucose, blood urea nitrogen (BUN), creatinine, coagulation studies, liver function tests (LFTs), and arterial (or venous) blood gas measurements to determine serum pH.

2. Plain abdominal radiographs should be obtained to assess for the presence of pills and to aid in monitoring bowel decontamination.

IV. TREATMENT

A. Advanced life support measures should be instituted as necessary.

1. Volume resuscitation with crystalloid is critically important in symptomatic patients.

2. Patients with signs of hypovolemia or acidosis require admission to the intensive care unit.

3. Individuals with mild symptoms require serial laboratory analysis and physical examination to evaluate ongoing GI absorption and the development of systemic toxicity.

4. Patients who remain or become asymptomatic at 6 hours after exposure may be discharged or referred to psychiatry in the case of intentional overdose.

B. Whole bowel irrigation (WBI; see Chapter 1) is the modality of choice for GI decontamination. Gastrotomy should be considered for the removal of large masses of iron from the gut when significant absorption continues despite WBI.

1. Activated charcoal is ineffective for binding charcoal, although it may be used for coingestions (see Chapter 1).

2. Emetics, gastric lavage, and cathartics are unlikely to result in significant iron removal.

C. Iron elimination can be enhanced by chelation with deferoxamine mesylate. Deferoxamine binds with iron to form a ferrioxamine complex that is excreted renally.

1. Treatment should not be delayed pending a serum iron concentration test in patients with clinical signs of serious poisoning (hypovolemia, GI bleeding, acidosis).

2. Chelation is indicated for an iron level over 500 µg/dL in the presence of lesser symptoms.
3. The deferoxamine challenge test (administering deferoxamine and looking for *vin-rosé*–colored urine resulting from the presence of ferrioxamine) is no longer recommended because it is not a sensitive indicator of toxicity.
4. Deferoxamine should be administered intravenously at a dose of 15 mg/kg/hour.
   a. The dose should be slowly increased to that rate over 30 minutes to avoid hypotension.
   b. Serum iron concentrations may be falsely lowered during the infusion.
5. Treatment should continue until the patient clinically improves and acidosis resolves. If the urine turns *vin rosé* color in response to the initial infusion, some authors recommend following urine samples as another end point for therapy (when color reverts to normal).
   a. Typically infusions are not needed beyond 12 to 24 hours.
   b. Treatment exceeding 24 to 48 hours is associated with pulmonary injury (acute respiratory distress syndrome, or ARDS) and nephrotoxicity.
   c. If patients require prolonged treatment, consideration should be given to a 12-hour hiatus each day.
6. Patients with renal failure may require dialysis to remove the ferrioxamine complex.
7. Pregnancy is not a contraindication to deferoxamine therapy.

V. COMPLICATIONS

A. GI bleeding, hepatitis, and coagulopathy should be treated by standard measures.
B. GI obstruction may require surgical intervention.

Selected Readings

Chyka PA, Butler AY. Assessment of acute iron poisoning by laboratory and clinical observations. *Am J Emerg Med* 1993 Mar;11:99–103.
This article discusses the utility of surrogate markers for the prediction of significant toxicity following iron overdose.

Mills KC, Curry SC. Acute iron poisoning. *Emerg Med Clin North Am* 1994 May;12: 397–413.
This in-depth review discusses the presentation and management of acute iron poisoning.

Palatnick W, Tenenbein M. Leukocytosis, hyperglycemia, vomiting, and positive x-rays are not indicators of severity of iron overdose in adults. *Am J Emerg Med* 1996 Sep;14:454–455.
Like the Chyka and Butler article, this one discusses the utility of surrogate markers for the prediction of significant toxicity following iron overdose.

Yatscoff RW, Wayne EA, Tenenbein M. An objective criterion for the cessation of deferoxamine therapy in the acutely iron poisoned patient. *J Toxicol Clin Toxicol* 1991; 29:431.
This article provides a rational approach for the discontinuation of deferoxamine therapy based on patient clinical condition.

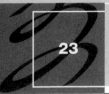

23 ISONIAZID POISONING
Steven B. Bird

I. BACKGROUND

A. Isoniazid (INH) is primarily used for the treatment of tuberculosis (TB).

B. INH overdose is most common in the American Indian population in Alaska and in the Southwest, where the prevalence of tuberculosis and the suicide rates are high.

C. It also occurs in urban areas where large populations of Southeast Asian and other third-world–country immigrants live.

II. PATHOPHYSIOLOGY

A. INH is rapidly and completely absorbed after oral administration, with peak concentrations normally occurring within 1 to 2 hours.

B. INH is widely distributed throughout the body with a volume of distribution approximating that of total body water (0.6 L/kg).

C. Most INH is metabolized in the liver within 24 hours by acetylation to acetylisoniazid and by hydrolysis to isonicotinic acid and hydrazine.

    1. Genetic variation in acetylation rate affects plasma concentration, elimination half-life, and toxicity.

    2. The elimination half-life is 0.5 to 1.5 hours in rapid acetylators and 2 to 4 hours in slow acetylators.

    3. Slow acetylators have increased concentrations of acetylhydrazine and hydrazine metabolites, which can cause hepatotoxicity.

    4. Advanced age, alcohol consumption, and rifampin coadministration can increase the risk of hepatotoxicity.

D. The usual therapeutic dose of INH is 5 mg/kg/day for adults and 10 mg/kg/day for children (up to a maximum of 300 mg/day).

E. Neurologic toxicity of INH is caused by its effects on γ-aminobutyric acid (GABA) glutamate concentrations in the brain.

    1. GABA is the primary inhibitory neurotransmitter, whereas glutamate is an excitatory neurotransmitter.

    2. The enzyme L-glutamic acid decarboxylase (GAD) converts glutamic acid to GABA with the active form of vitamin B_6 (pyridoxal $5L$-phosphate) acting as coenzyme.

    3. INH decreases GABA synthesis by:

        a. lowering vitamin B_6 (pyridoxine) concentrations in the body through the formation of INH–pyridoxine hydrazones.

        b. competitively inhibiting the conversion of pyridoxine to pyridoxal $5'$ phosphate.

    c. inactivating pyridoxal phosphate-containing enzymes.

  4. Acute ingestion of 1.5 to 3 g in adults is potentially toxic, and 6 to 10 g can cause severe poisoning.

  5. In patients with epilepsy, seizures have occurred with doses as low as 14 mg/kg/day.

F. Metabolic acidosis results from lactic acidosis secondary to seizure activity and interference with nicotinamide-adenine dinucleotide (NAD)–mediated conversion of lactate to pyruvate.

G. Hyperglycemia results from inhibition of specific steps in the Krebs cycle that require NAD and from stimulation of glucagon secretion.

H. INH-induced hepatitis may be caused by the covalent binding of hydrazine metabolites to liver macromolecules.

I. Peripheral neuropathy associated with INH therapy results from pyridoxine deficiency.

III. DIAGNOSIS

A. Clinical Toxicity

  1. Effects appear 30 minutes to 2 hours after acute overdose.

  2. Nausea, vomiting, dizziness, slurred speech, blurred vision, and visual hallucinations are among the first symptoms.

  3. Lethargy, stupor, and coma can develop rapidly, followed by tonic–clonic seizures and hyperreflexia or areflexia.

  4. In severe cases, cardiovascular and respiratory collapse can result in death.

  5. Metabolic abnormalities include severe metabolic acidosis, hyperglycemia, hyperkalemia, glycosuria, and ketonuria.

  6. The triad of metabolic acidosis refractory to sodium bicarbonate therapy, seizures refractory to anticonvulsants, and coma suggests INH overdose.

  7. Hepatotoxicity from chronic exposure is usually manifested by elevated serum aminotransferase concentrations within the first few months of therapy.

  8. Peripheral neuropathy can occur anytime during therapy.

B. Differential Diagnosis

  1. Other toxic causes of seizures include carbon monoxide, cyanide, camphor, cocaine, cyclic antidepressants, hydrazine, propoxyphene, sympathomimetics, salicylates, theophylline, and withdrawal states.

  2. Central nervous system infection, hemorrhage, and trauma should also be considered in the differential diagnosis.

C. Evaluation

  1. Laboratory evaluation should include blood glucose, electrolyte, blood urea nitrogen (BUN), creatinine, liver profile, and arterial blood gas determinations and urine toxicological screening.

  2. Patients with coma or seizures should have a chest x-ray and electrocardiogram (ECG). Cranial computed tomography should be performed in those with neurologic symptoms that are unresponsive to antidotal therapy.

IV. TREATMENT

A. Advanced life support measures should be instituted as necessary.

B. Gastrointestinal decontamination with activated charcoal should be considered for recent overdose (see Chapter 1).

C. Pyridoxine or vitamin B_6 is considered the antidote for neurologic toxicity.

    1. It can reverse coma as well as prevent and terminate seizures, which leads to the resolution of metabolic acidosis.

    2. A dose of pyridoxine equal to the amount of INH ingested should be given at the first sign of neurologic toxicity.

        a. If the amount ingested is not known, at least 5 g of parenteral pyridoxine should be given.

        b. It should be given as a bolus over 3 to 5 minutes in those with seizures.

        c. In patients without seizure activity, pyridoxine can be administered intravenously (IV) over 30 minutes.

        d. Peripheral neuropathy related to pyridoxine deficiency can be prevented by coadministration of oral pyridoxine.

D. Seizures should also be treated with benzodiazepines. Diazepam has been shown to potentiate the action of pyridoxine.

E. IV sodium bicarbonate should be given to correct acidemia, but it is not very effective until seizures are terminated.

F. Hemodialysis or hemoperfusion should be considered in patients with intractable acid-base abnormalities, persistent seizures, and liver or renal failure.

V. COMPLICATIONS

A. Complications include rhabdomyolysis, renal failure, and aspiration pneumonia.

B. Severe acidemia can result in cardiovascular collapse and multiple-organ failure.

Selected Readings

Bredemann JA, Krechel SW, Eggers GWN. Treatment of refractory seizures in massive isoniazid overdose. *Anesth Analg* 1990;71:554–557.
A discussion of the pathophysiology of INH-induced seizures and pyridoxine therapy as well as use of thiopental infusion for refractory seizures.

Brent J, Vo N, Kulig K, et al. Reversal of prolonged isoniazid-induced coma by pyridoxine. *Arch Intern Med* 1990;150:1751–1753.
Three case reports and discussion on the effectiveness of pyridoxine in reversing INH-induced coma.

Chin L, Sievers ML, Laird HE, et al. Evaluation of diazepam and pyridoxine as antidotes to isoniazid intoxication in rats and dogs. *Toxicol Appl Pharmacol* 1978;45:713–722.
Basic science evidence to support the concomitant use of pyridoxine and diazepam in preventing INH-induced seizures and coma.

Dickinson DS, Bailey WC, Hirschowitz BI, et al. Risk factors for isoniazid (INH)-induced liver dysfunction. *J Clin Gastroenterol* 1981;3:271–279.
A prospective review of risk factors for isoniazid-induced liver dysfunction, suggesting slow acetylators seem to be at increased risk.

Konigshausen TH, Altrogge G, Hein D, et al. Hemodialysis and hemoperfusion in the treatment of most severe INH poisoning. *Vet Hum Toxicol* 1979;21(Suppl): 12–15.
A discussion of two cases of INH poisoning treated with hemodialysis and hemoperfusion.

Wason S, Lacouture PG, Lovejoy FH. Single high-dose pyridoxine treatment for isoniazid overdose. *JAMA* 1981;246:1102–1104.
A review of clinical outcomes of patients treated with high-dose pyridoxine therapy versus little or no pyridoxine, demonstrating pyridoxine's beneficial effects in terminating seizures and lessening coma.

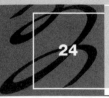

24 LITHIUM
D. Eric Brush

I. BACKGROUND

A. Lithium is primarily used for the treatment of bipolar and unipolar depression.

B. It is available as 300 mg immediate-release and 450 mg sustained-release lithium carbonate tablets (8 and 12 mEq lithium, respectively) and a citrate solution (8 mEq lithium per 5 mL).

C. Therapeutic serum concentrations are 0.8 to 1.25 mEq/L.

II. PATHOPHYSIOLOGY

A. Lithium competes with Na^+ for ion transport, enhances serotonin and acetylcholine effects, and acts as an inhibitory second messenger via inositol phosphates.

B. Oral absorption of immediate-release formulations is complete within 1 to 6 hours. Peak serum concentrations occur 2 to 4 hours after therapeutic doses.

C. Absorption is prolonged with sustained-release preparations and with overdose. Peak serum concentration may be delayed up to 48 hours after overdose.

D. Distribution is slow and biphasic.

  1. Lithium initially distributes in extracellular fluid with a volume distribution of 0.3 to 0.4 L/kg.

  2. It then distributes into tissue with final volume distribution of 0.7 to 1 L/kg.

  3. Serum lithium levels do not reflect tissue levels until 10 to 12 hours after a therapeutic dose and longer after overdose.

  4. As a result of slow distribution, high serum concentrations without significant toxicity may initially be seen following overdose, and toxicity may later develop as serum levels decline.

  5. Lithium is not bound to serum proteins and crosses the placenta freely.

E. Elimination occurs almost exclusively by renal excretion, with small amounts eliminated in sweat, feces, and breast milk.

  1. Renal tubular reabsorption is increased in sodium-depleted states.

    a. Dehydration from sweating, gastrointestinal (GI) losses, or diuretics leads to increased lithium reabsorption.

    b. Renal failure from dehydration or drugs such as nonsteroidal antiinflammatory drugs (NSAIDs) also leads to decreased lithium excretion.

2. The half-life after a single dose is about 24 hours but can be as long as 48 hours with chronic therapy.

III. DIAGNOSIS

A. Clinical Presentation

1. Acute overdose of more than 1 mEq/kg (40 mg/kg lithium carbonate) can cause toxicity.

2. Chronic toxicity is usually the result of a condition that decreases renal lithium excretion.

3. Acute toxicity tends to cause an early predominance of GI symptoms followed later by central nervous system (CNS) symptoms, whereas an individual with chronic toxicity generally presents with altered mental status but without GI symptoms.

4. Manifestations of mild toxicity include nausea, vomiting, lethargy, fatigue, memory impairment, and fine tremor.

5. Moderate toxicity is characterized by confusion, agitation, delirium, coarse tremor, hyperreflexia, hypertension, tachycardia, dysarthria, nystagmus, ataxia, muscle fasciculations, extrapyramidal symptoms, and choreoathetoid movements.

6. With severe toxicity, bradycardia, coma, seizures, hyperthermia, and hypotension can be seen.

7. In chronic poisoning, mild toxicity is associated with lithium levels less than 1.5 mEq/L, moderate toxicity with levels of 1.5 to 3.0 mEq/L, and severe toxicity with levels of more than 3.0 mEq/L.

8. Because of slow distribution, levels following acute overdose do not initially correlate with clinical toxicity.

9. Findings that can be seen with both therapeutic and toxic drug levels include:

a. Nonspecific electrocardiographic (ECG) changes such as U waves; flat, biphasic, or inverted T waves; and, rarely, sinus or junctional bradycardia or sinoatrial (SA) or atrioventricular (AV) nodal block.

b. Leukocytosis

c. Nephrogenic diabetes insipidus (lack of response to vasopressin) with dilute urine and elevated sodium, blood urea nitrogen (BUN), and creatinine.

B. Differential Diagnosis

1. Nausea and vomiting may be mistakenly attributed to GI conditions.

2. The differential diagnosis of neuromuscular symptoms includes hypoglycemia, hypoxia, infection, stroke, hypercalcemia, hyperthyroidism, and the serotonin syndrome (see Chapter 7)

C. Evaluation

1. All patients taking lithium who develop an intercurrent illness causing decreased fluid intake or increased fluid losses should have their lithium level measured.

2. Evaluation of patients with potential lithium poisoning should also include a complete blood count (CBC), serum electrolytes, BUN, creatinine, glucose, calcium, magnesium, and an ECG.

3. After acute overdose, serum lithium levels should be repeated every 4 hours until a peak is observed.

IV. TREATMENT

A. Advanced life support measures should be instituted as necessary.

B. Volume replacement with intravenous (IV) normal saline with the goal of establishing a brisk urine output (1 to 3 mL/kg/h) should be instituted in all symptomatic patients.

1. This allows normal renal clearance of lithium: 15 to 30 mL/min.

2. Follow serum electrolytes for hypernatremia.

C. IV dextrose, naloxone, and thiamine should be considered for those with altered mental status.

D. Benzodiazepines should be given for seizures.

E. Cooling measures should be instituted for patients with hyperthermia.

F. Although activated charcoal is ineffective for binding lithium, it should be considered if coingestants are suspected (see Chapter 1).

G. Whole bowel irrigation (see Chapter 1) should be considered for patients with persistently rising lithium levels, and particularly for those with sustained-release preparation overdose.

H. Hemodialysis is the most efficient method of enhancing the elimination of lithium, with clearances of 100 to 300 mL/min.

1. Indications for hemodialysis include:

   a. Significant neurologic dysfunction (e.g, confusion, inability to walk) along with an elevated lithium concentration.

   b. Chronic toxicity with lithium concentration greater than 3 mEq/L.

   c. Acute ingestion with peak lithium level greater than 9 to 10 mEq/L, because significant toxicity is likely to develop after distribution (some advocate dialysis for concentrations greater than 4 mEq/L and rising in acute poisoning).

   d. Moderate clinical toxicity and renal failure (owing to inability to eliminate lithium) or congestive heart failure, pulmonary edema, cerebral edema, or anasarca (owing to inability to tolerate saline hydration).

2. Dialysis (intermittent or continuous) should be continued until the lithium level is less than 1 mEq/L.

3. Serum lithium level should be checked 6 hours after dialysis to detect possible rebound increase in level as redistribution occurs.

I. Amiloride is effective for the treatment of lithium-induced diabetes insipidus.

V. COMPLICATIONS

A. Permanent sequelae such as encephalopathy, choreoathetosis, nystagmus, and ataxia can result from moderate or severe poisoning.

B. Whether enhanced elimination therapy can prevent such complications is unknown.

Suggested Readings

Jaeger A, Sauder P, Kopfersehmitt J, et al. When should dialysis be performed in lithium poisoning? A kinetic study in 14 cases of lithium poisoning. *J Toxicol Clin Toxicol* 1993;31:429–447.
A study on lithium kinetics suggesting criteria for and timing of dialysis.

Smith SW, Ling LJ, Halstenson CE. Whole-bowel irrigation as a treatment for acute lithium overdose. *Ann Emerg Med* 1991;20:536–539.
A human volunteer study showing the effectiveness of whole bowel irrigation for enhancing lithium decontamination.

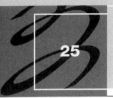

25 LOCAL ANESTHETICS
Ivan E. Liang

I. BACKGROUND

  A. Local anesthetics (Table 25-1) are a class of drugs originally based on the chemistry of cocaine that are used to produce regions of analgesia.
  B. They are introduced transdermally as creams or sprays, or by local needle infiltration, into specific anatomic plains (epidurals), or intravenously (IV; Bier block).
  C. Toxicity typically results either from adverse side effects (allergic reactions, methemoglobinemia), iatrogenic overdose, or from accidental intravascular infusion.

II. PATHOPHYSIOLOGY

  A. Local anesthetics work predominantly by reversibly binding to and inhibiting membrane sodium channels.
  B. Pain and temperature sensation are most affected because of the small diameter of their nerve fibers.
  C. Inhibition of sodium channels in excitable cells of the central nervous system (CNS) and the myocardium is responsible for systemic toxicity, although other mechanisms exist.
    1. Bupivacaine has been shown to impair mitochondrial oxidative phosphorylation.
    2. High concentrations of local anesthetics may also be directly cytotoxic to neurons.
  D. Systemic toxicity is closely related to plasma drug concentrations, with minor CNS symptoms (lightheadedness) proceeding to major CNS symptoms (seizure), and subsequent myocardial depression and dysrhythmias.
    1. Maximal recommended doses for local infiltration include 300 mg of lidocaine, 400 mg of bupivacaine, 15 mg of tetracaine, and 600 mg of procaine.
    2. Toxicity is typically associated with single-dose IV exposure of 6.4 mg of lidocaine, 1.6 mg of bupivacaine, 2.5 mg of tetracaine, or 19.2 mg of procaine.
  E. Allergic reactions are very rare and predominantly associated with amino ester agents (Table 25-1), which are rapidly metabolized by plasma cholinesterase to paraaminobenzoic acid (PABA), a well-known allergen. Some multidose preparations of amino amide agents contain methylparaben, another known allergen.

TABLE 25-1	Systemic Local Anesthetics Available in the United States

Esters
   Chloroprocaine (Nesacaine)
   Procaine (Novocain)
   Tetracaine (Pontocaine)
Amides
   Mepivacaine (Carbocaine)
   Etidocaine (Duranest)
   Bupivacaine (Marcaine, Sensorcaine)
   Ropivacaine (Naropin)
   Lidocaine (Xylocaine)

Source: Irwin RS, Rippe JM. *Manual of Intensive Care Medicine,*
3rd ed. Philadelphia: Lippincott Williams & Wilkins, 2000:639.

F. Methemoglobinemia is most commonly reported as a side effect of topical benzocaine exposure as a result of oxidizing metabolites, but it can result from large exposures of the other agents (notably prilocaine).

III. DIAGNOSIS

A. Clinical Toxicity
    1. Onset is generally very rapid because of the nature of exposure (intramuscular or intravascular).
    2. Minor symptoms include perioral and tongue numbness, lightheadedness, and visual and auditory disturbances including frank psychosis.
    3. More severe effects include depressed level of consciousness, coma, seizures, and cardiovascular depression.
        a. Hypotension is the result of decreased cardiac output and dysrhythmias.
        b. Blockade of sodium channels results in prolongation of PR and QRS intervals (see Chapter 5).
        c. At high plasma levels, sinus arrest with junctional rhythms and atrioventricular (AV) block can occur.
        d. Cardiovascular effects are potentiated by acidosis, hypoxia, and hypercarbia.
    4. Methemoglobinemia typically causes dyspnea, cyanosis, and symptoms of hypoxia with dual-wave pulse oximetry measures of 85% (see Chapter 34).

B. Evaluation
    1. Evaluation should include cardiac monitoring, an electrocardiogram, and testing for serum electrolytes.
    2. The methemoglobin fraction should be measured in patients with cyanosis or symptoms of hypoxia (see Chapter 34). A careful history should be taken in patients presenting with methemoglobinemia in

regard to benzocaine exposure, which is found in pediatric teething powders and adult throat sprays.
3. Except for lidocaine, serum drug levels are rarely available soon enough to be of clinical use.
   a. Serum lidocaine levels of 5 to 10 mg/L are associated with minor CNS effects.
   b. Levels of 10 to 20 mg/L are associated with major CNS effects.
   c. Levels greater than 20 mg/L are associated with cardiorespiratory arrest.

C. Differential Diagnosis
1. Clinical situations in which toxicity develops are usually apparent and in close relation to a procedure involving one of these agents.
2. Care must be given to distinguish early CNS toxicity from anxiety or vasovagal reactions to a procedure.

IV. TREATMENT

A. Advanced life support measures should be instituted as necessary.
B. Seizures can be treated with benzodiazepines and barbiturates. They should be rapidly controlled so as to prevent further acidemia.
C. Hypotension should be treated with IV fluids followed by pressor agents such as norepinephrine.
D. Bradydysrhythmias should be treated with atropine.
   1. They (especially from bupivacaine) are notoriously refractory to standard advanced cardiac life support (ACLS) protocols.
   2. Amrinone has been found to be effective in animal models.
   3. Other agents that have been used but are of unclear benefit include bretylium, phenytoin, magnesium, amiodarone, and dobutamine.
E. Factors that potentiate toxicity, such as acidosis, hypoxemia, and hyperkalemia, should be corrected.
F. End-organ perfusion may need to be supported by balloon pumping or cardiopulmonary bypass.
G. Hemoperfusion may be of benefit in decreasing plasma levels.
H. Allergic reactions should be managed as for allergic reactions from other causes.
I. Methemoglobinemia is treated with oxygen and methylene blue (see Chapter 35).

Suggested Readings
Naguib M, Magboul MM, Samarkandi AH, et al. Adverse effects and drug interactions associated with local and regional anaesthesia. *Drug Saf* 1998 Apr;18(4):221–250.
This article reviews the adverse reactions, interactions, and toxicity of local anesthetics.

Reiz S, Nath S. Cardiotoxicity of local anaesthetic agents. *Br J Anaesth* 1986;58: 736–746.
This article summarizes the cardiovascular toxicity of local anesthetics.

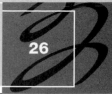

I. BACKGROUND

A. Theophylline is the methylxanthine of most clinical importance, although caffeine and theobromine (with similar clinical toxicity) may also be encountered.

B. Intentional overdoses and dosing errors (e.g., miscalculation of dose, change in frequency of administration, lack of serum drug level monitoring, unrecognized drug interaction leading to reduced clearance of theophylline) account for most poisonings.

II. PATHOPHYSIOLOGY

A. Although the pathophysiology of theophylline remains incompletely understood, three primary mechanisms have been postulated:

  1. Inhibition of cyclic guanosine monophosphate (cGMP) or adenosine monophosphate (cAMP) activity.

  2. Adenosine receptor antagonism.

  3. β-Adrenergic stimulation secondary to elevated levels of circulating plasma catecholamines.

B. Theophylline is metabolized by the CYP-450 mixed-function oxidase system in the liver.

C. Many drugs, chemicals, and medical conditions affect the steady-state serum concentration and elimination half-life of theophylline.

  1. Drugs or conditions increasing serum theophylline concentration include erythromycin, fluoroquinolones, cimetidine, β-blockers, cirrhosis, and congestive heart failure (CHF).

  2. At therapeutic doses, the elimination half-life of theophylline varies widely with the age of the patient.

   a. The half-life averages 4.5 to 5 hours in healthy adults.

   b. It is shorter in children and smokers (induced metabolism).

   c. It is longer in infants, the elderly, and those with heart, liver, and pulmonary disease.

III. DIAGNOSIS

A. Clinical Toxicity

  1. Theophylline toxicity is characterized by cardiac, central nervous system (CNS), gastrointestinal (GI), and musculoskeletal symptoms as well as metabolic derangements.

2. Sinus tachycardia is invariably present, but supraventricular tachycardia and ventricular arrhythmias can also occur.
3. In mild theophylline poisoning, mild hypertension can occur, whereas in severe theophylline poisoning, hypotension with a widened pulse pressure is seen.
4. Seizures are also characteristic of severe theophylline poisoning.
   a. They are usually recurrent and resistant to conventional anticonvulsants and can be focal.
   b. They are associated with a high frequency of permanent neurologic disability and a mortality rate that approaches 50% in elderly patients.
5. GI effects include vomiting, diarrhea, and hematemesis.
6. Skeletal muscle tremor, a common feature, can include myoclonic jerks.
7. Metabolic disturbances include acidosis, hypokalemia, hyperglycemia, hypophosphatemia, hypomagnesemia, and hypercalcemia. Hypokalemia results from the intracellular shift of potassium rather than from decreased total body potassium content.
8. Effects depend on whether the poisoning occurs through a single ingestion (acute intoxication), chronic overmedication (chronic intoxication), or acute or therapeutic intoxication.
9. After acute overdose, mild clinical intoxication (nausea, vomiting, tachycardia) occurs with theophylline concentrations of 20 to 40 μg/mL; with levels greater than 70 μg/ml, life-threatening events (intractable seizures and severe cardiac arrhythmias) can appear.
10. Metabolic abnormalities are seen more commonly with acute intoxications.
11. In chronic intoxication, no correlation is seen between serum theophylline concentration and the appearance of life-threatening events.
    a. Age under 6 months or over 60 years is a risk factor.
    b. Serious toxicity can occur even with theophylline concentrations in the therapeutic or mildly toxic range.
12. Toxicity is typically delayed and prolonged after overdose with sustained-release formulations.

B. Evaluation

1. Laboratory tests should include serum theophylline concentration, electrolytes, blood urea nitrogen (BUN), creatinine, calcium, magnesium, phosphorus, glucose, and creatine phosphokinase (CPK), complete blood count (CBC), urinalysis (for evidence of myoglobinuria), and electrocardiogram (ECG).
2. Arterial blood gases and a chest x-ray should be obtained for patients with severe poisoning.
3. Theophylline concentrations should be obtained every 1 to 2 hours until a peak or plateau and subsequent decline has been observed.

IV. TREATMENT

A. Advanced life support measures should be instituted as necessary. Supportive care should focus on airway protection, correction of cardiovascular abnormalities, and maintenance of normal blood pH.

B. Oral activated charcoal (see Chapter 1) is highly effective in reducing the absorption of theophylline and should be administered to virtually all patients with theophylline toxicity.

C. Adenosine can be used to treat hemodynamically significant supraventricular tachycardia.

D. Lidocaine is the recommended treatment for ventricular arrhythmias with hemodynamic compromise.

E. Hypotension should be treated with intravenous (IV) fluids and an IV β-blocker (propranolol 1 to 2 mg IV or a continuous esmolol infusion).

F. Norepinephrine may be more efficacious than dopamine for persistent hypotension.

G. Seizures should be treated with high doses of benzodiazepines.
   1. Phenytoin is unlikely to be effective.
   2. Thiopental or pentobarbital may be necessary for prolonged seizures.
   3. Neuromuscular blockade should also be considered for refractory seizures because of potential morbidity resulting from rhabdomyolysis, hyperthermia, and acidosis.

H. Hypokalemia is best treated by lowering the theophylline concentration. Aggressive potassium replacement can result in hyperkalemia when toxicity resolves.

I. Multiple-dose activated charcoal (see Chapter 1) greatly enhances the elimination of theophylline and can be as effective as hemodialysis.
   1. Aggressive antiemetic therapy including metoclopramide (up to 1 mg/kg IV per dose) and a serotonin antagonist such as ondansetron may be necessary for the patient to tolerate charcoal.
   2. Cimetidine should be avoided because it impairs theophylline clearance.

J. In severely intoxicated patients, consultation with a nephrologist and rapid removal of theophylline using hemodialysis or hemoperfusion are imperative (Table 26-1).
   1. Indications for extracorporeal drug removal should be liberalized in patients with respiratory failure, CHF, or liver disease.
   2. Charcoal hemoperfusion is more effective in removing theophylline than hemodialysis is, but hemodialysis is more readily performed and more widely available and has a lower risk of bleeding diathesis.

TABLE 26-1	**Indications for Hemodialysis/Hemoperfusion**

Acute poisoning
Peak serum theophylline concentration >80–100 μg/mL
Peak serum theophylline concentration >60–80 μg/mL and intractable vomiting
Theophylline concentration >70 μg/mL 4 hours after ingestion of sustained-release preparation
Seizures, cardiac arrhythmias, or hypotension and theophylline concentration >40 μg/mL
Chronic poisoning
Age >60 years or <6 months and theophylline concentration >40 μg/mL
Age <60 years or >6 months and theophylline concentration >60 μg/mL

V. COMPLICATIONS

A. Complications include pulmonary aspiration and rhadomyolysis.

B. Persistent encephalopathy has been reported in patients with seizures.

Selected Readings

Amitai Y, Lovejoy FH. Characteristics of vomiting associated with acute sustained release theophylline poisoning: implications for management with oral activated charcoal. *J Toxicol Clin Toxicol* 1987;25:539–554.
   A case series of patients with protracted vomiting from acute theophylline toxicity and limited ability to tolerate oral charcoal, suggesting the need for aggressive antiemetic therapy.

Olson KR, Benowitz NL, Woo OF, et al. Theophylline overdose: acute single ingestion versus chronic repeated overmedication. *Am J Emerg Med* 1985;3:386–394.
   A case series of patients with acute and chronic theophylline intoxication demonstrating different clinical and metabolic characteristics between the two groups.

Shannon M. Life-threatening events after theophylline overdose: a 10-year prospective analysis. *Arch Intern Med* 1999;159:989–994.
   Most comprehensive series of patients with theophylline intoxication demonstrating that chronic overmedication results in significantly more morbidity and mortality.

Shannon M. Predictors of major toxicity after theophylline overdose. *Ann Intern Med* 1993;119:1161–1167.
   A prospective series of 249 patients demonstrating that major toxicity was associated with peak theophylline concentration greater than 100 mg/L after acute intoxication and age more than 60 years (regardless of theophylline concentration) after chronic overmedication.

Shannon M, Lovejoy FH. The influence of age vs. peak serum concentration on life-threatening events after chronic theophylline intoxication. *Arch Intern Med* 1990; 150:2045–2048.
   A case series of patients with chronic theophylline intoxication demonstrating that peak theophylline concentration was not predictive of which patients would have seizures or arrhythmias.

Shannon MW. Comparative efficacy of hemodialysis and hemoperfusion in severe theophylline intoxication. *Acad Emerg Med* 1997;4:674–678.
   A 10-year prospective observational study demonstrating comparable efficacy of hemodialysis and hemoperfusion in reducing the morbidity of severe theophylline intoxication.

I. BACKGROUND

A. Neuromuscular blockers (NMBs) are used to facilitate intubation and airway control, decrease oxygen consumption, improve compliance with mechanical ventilation refractory to sedatives, and abolish excessive muscular contractions that may lead to hyperthermia and rhabdomyolysis.

B. NMBs are structurally similar to acetylcholine and are categorized as nondepolarizing or depolarizing agents.

C. Nondepolarizing NMBs include pancuronium, vecuronium, atracurium, rocuronium, and *d*-tubocurarine.

D. Succinylcholine is the only depolarizing NMB in common use.

II. PATHOPHYSIOLOGY

A. Nondepolarizing NMBs compete with acetylcholine at receptor sites.

 1. On the motor endplate, they prevent depolarization and contraction of skeletal muscle fibers.

 2. They also block presynaptic receptors, which can prevent positive feedback and decrease the production of acetylcholine.

B. Succinylcholine acts similarly to acetylcholine at the endplate receptor, causing persistent depolarization of the postjunctional membrane.

 1. This causes initial muscle fasciculation followed by paralysis.

 2. Paralysis occurs because succinylcholine is not metabolized as rapidly as acetylcholine is, and the depolarized membrane remains unresponsive to additional impulses.

C. The pharmacologic properties of NMBs make them more or less useful for specific patients and clinical situations (Table 27-1).

 1. The time to onset of paralysis for each drug, which is determined by dose, distribution and redistribution kinetics, and receptor sensitivity, generally occurs within 3 to 5 minutes.

 2. Elimination varies by route of metabolism and excretion.

 3. Despite similar plasma concentrations and dosing techniques, intensity and duration of neuromuscular blockade vary from patient to patient.

 4. Succinylcholine is used primarily for rapid-sequence intubation because of an unpredictable duration of action with prolonged use.

 5. Rocuronium is a comparable short-acting, nondepolarizing NMB.

TABLE 27-1 — Pharmacology Summary of Selected Neuromuscular Blockers

Drug	Onset	Duration	Metabolism	Elimination
Depolarizing				
Succinylcholine	0.5–1 min	4–6 min	Plasma cholinesterases	10% unchanged in urine
Nondepolarizing				
Long-acting				
Pancuronium	2–3 min	30–60 min	30% to 40% by liver	60% unchanged drug and metabolites in urine, 11% in bile
Intermediate-acting				
Vecuronium	2–5 min	20–40 min	Spontaneous deacetylation and liver metabolism, active metabolites	20% unchanged drug in urine, 45% unchanged drug, and 25% metabolites in bile
Atracurium	3–5 min	20–35 min	Ester hydrolysis and Hofmann elimination in plasma	Unchanged drug and metabolites in urine and bile
Short-acting				
Mivacurium	3–5 min	15–30 min	Ester hydrolysis by plasma and cholinesterase in plasma	Unchanged drug and metabolites in urine and bile
Rocuronium	1 min	30–60 min	Deacetylation and liver metabolism, inactive metabolite	Primarily biliary excretion, 33% unchanged drug in urine

Source: Irwin RS, Rippe JM. *Manual of Intensive Care Medicine*, 3rd ed. Philadelphia: Lippincott Williams & Wilkins, 2000:660.

TABLE 27-2	Dosing Guidelines for Selected Neuromuscular Blockage Agents

| Drug | Single/intermittent dose | Continuous infusion | |
		Loading dose	Maintenance dose
Succinylcholine	1–2 mg/kg	N/A	N/A
Rocuronium	0.8 mg/kg	N/A	N/A
Pancuronium	0.1–0.2 mg/kg every 1–3 hrs	0.03–0.1 mg/kg	0.06–0.1 mg/kg/h
Vecuronium	0.1–0.2 mg/kg every 1 hr	0.1 mg/kg	0.05–0.1 mg/kg/h
Atracurium	0.5 mg/kg	0.5 mg/kg	0.4–1.0 mg/kg/h

Source: Irwin RS, Rippe JM. *Manual of Intensive Care Medicine,* 3rd ed. Philadelphia: Lippincott Williams & Wilkins, 2000:661.

D. Dosing should be individualized and based on lean body weight (Table 27-2).

   1. Longer-acting NMBs (pancuronium and vecuronium) are usually administered by intermittent bolus as needed to achieve clinical goals.

   2. Intermittent bolus therapy is impractical for prolonged therapy with shorter-acting NMBs such as atracurium or rocuronium.

   3. Continuous infusion of NMBs may reduce required daily dosages compared with intermittent bolus therapy.

   4. Infusion rates should be titrated based on individual response.

   5. Reduced doses may be appropriate for patients with renal and hepatic dysfunction, particularly the elderly.

   a. Because of pancuronium's primary renal clearance, a reduction in dosing of up to 50% may be required for patients with renal dysfunction.

   b. Infusions of vecuronium may need to be reduced by 50% in patients with cholestasis and hepatic dysfunction.

   c. Dose reduction in patients with renal and hepatic dysfunction is not required with atracurium.

   6. Hyperdynamic patients (e.g., those with burns) may exhibit decreased sensitivity to competitive NMBs and require two to five times the normal dose.

   7. Increases in dosage requirements have also been described for critically ill patients receiving prolonged continuous infusions of NMBs, possibly because of changes in the neuromuscular junction causing drug resistance.

III. DIAGNOSIS

A. Adverse Effects

   1. Nonimmunologic histamine release from mast cells:

   a. Occurs with tubocurarine, atracurium, mivacurium, and succinylcholine.

b. Effects include venous and arterial dilation, hypotension, tachycardia, bronchospasm, and facial and upper body erythema.
2. Anaphylaxis/anaphylactoid reactions
  a. Occur very rarely.
  b. Most often are associated with succinylcholine.
3. Increased neuromuscular blockade results from:
  a. Anticholinesterase agents such as physostigmine, neostigmine, and carbamate and organophosphate insecticides.
  b. Aminoglycosides, which decrease acetylcholine release and stabilize postjunctional membranes.
  c. Cardiovascular agents such as β-blockers, calcium channel blockers, procainamide, furosemide, and quinidine.
  d. Genetic deficiency in plasma cholinesterase activity.
    (1) Succinycholine is predominantly hydrolyzed by plasma cholinesterase.
    (2) Mivacurium is also hydrolyzed by plasma cholinesterase.
4. Chronic anticonvulsant therapy can decrease neuromuscular blocking effects.
5. Hyperkalemia
  a. Serum potassium increases by 0.5 mEq/L for each mg/kg of succinylcholine administered.
  b. Severe hyperkalemia can occur in patients who have upregulated extrajunctional acetylcholine receptors, such as those with head or spinal cord injury, stroke, neuropathy, critical illness neuropathy or myopathy, muscular dystrophy, thermal burn or cold injury, crush injury, prolonged immobility, malignant hyperthermia, or prolonged exposure to nondepolarizing agents.
  c. Succinylcholine is typically not used for children because of the risk of undiagnosed muscular dystrophy.
7. Postparalytic syndromes
  a. Can occur with intermittent or short-term dosing regimens as well as with continuous infusions.
  b. Weakness without myopathy can persist for a few hours or days after termination of treatment.
  c. Myopathy (paresis, increased creatine phosphokinase [CPK], abnormal motor unit electromyography with normal sensory nerve conduction) with weakness lasting for several weeks to months can also occur.
  d. Causative or contributing factors include excessive NMB dosing, drug interactions, delayed elimination of parent drug or metabolites as a result of organ dysfunction, and metabolic derangements.
  e. Routinely discontinuing neuromuscular blockade and sedation for brief intervals on a daily basis may prevent postparalytic syndromes.
8. Malignant hyperthermia:
  a. May be triggered by exposure to volatile halogenated anesthetics and succinylcholine.
  b. Is characterized by hypermetabolism (hyperthermia, muscular rigidity, labile vital signs, lactic acidosis, hyperkalemia, rhabdomyolysis).
  c. Is caused by abnormal calcium release from the sarcoplasmic reticulum.

d. Susceptible patients have genetic predisposition or diseases such as Duchenne muscular dystrophy.
e. Drugs considered safe in such individuals include nondepolarizing NMBs, nitrous oxide, propofol, ketamine, etomidate, benzodiazepines, barbiturates, opioids, and local anesthetics.

B. Evaluation

1. Patients with prolonged weakness should have a complete blood count (CBC), serum electrolytes, blood urea nitrogen (BUN), creatinine, glucose, CPK, urinalysis, and electrocardiogram.
2. Use of train-of-four (TOF) peripheral nerve stimulation to monitor neuromuscular blockade and limiting the dose of NMB to that which blocks only one or two of four potential twitches may decrease the incidence and severity of prolonged paralysis.

IV. TREATMENT

A. Histamine reactions should be treated with H_1 and H_2 blockers.
B. Anaphylactic reactions and hyperkalemia should be treated with standard therapies.
C. Acetylcholinesterase inhibitors such as neostigmine, pyridostigmine, and edrophonium can reverse the effects of most nondepolarizing NMBs.
   1. Edrophonium acts faster than neostigmine and pyridostigmine do.
   2. Antimuscarinic agents are usually coadministered (atropine with edrophonium and glycopyrrolate with neostigmine and pyridostigmine) to minimize muscarinic receptor activation.
   3. Neostigmine and pyridostigmine, but not edrophonium, inhibit plasma cholinesterase and thus may potentiate the effects of mivacurium.
D. The treatment of malignant hyperthermia includes:
   1. Stopping the triggering agent.
   2. Administering dantrolene as a 2 to 3 mg/kg rapid intravenous bolus followed by additional doses until symptoms abate (up to 10 mg/kg total dose).
   3. Aggressive supportive care, with close attention to treating hyperthermia, acidosis, and hyperkalemia.

V. COMPLICATIONS

A. Adverse effects are described earlier.
B. Other complications of NMB therapy include stress resulting from failure to coadminister sedatives, ventilator mishaps, pressure-induced skin breakdown, rhabdomyolysis, peripheral neuropathy, deconditioning, and venous thromboembolism.

Selected Readings

Ali HH, Savarese JJ. Monitoring of neuromuscular function. *Anesthesiology* 1976;45: 216–249.
An excellent review of the pathophysiology of neuromuscular blockade and monitoring of neuromuscular function.

Fiamengo SA, Savarese JJ. Use of muscle relaxants in intensive care units. *Crit Care Med* 1991;19:1457–1459.
A succinct review of complications and adverse effects of neuromuscular relaxants and the need for monitoring with peripheral nerve stimulators.

Goldfrank LR, Flomenbaum N, Lewin N, et al. *Goldfrank's Toxicologic Emergencies,* 7th ed. McGraw-Hill, New York, 2002:806–823.
An excellent overview of the clinically relevant agents.

Gooch JL, Suchyta MR, Balbierz JM, et al. Prolonged paralysis after treatment with neuromuscular junction blocking agents. *Crit Care Med* 1991;19:1125–1131.
A case series of intensive care unit patients with prolonged paralysis after treatment with neuromuscular blocking agents, demonstrating neurogenic atrophy based on electrodiagnostic and muscle pathology findings.

Larijani GE, Gratz I, Silverberg M, et al. Clinical pharmacology of the neuromuscular blocking agents. *DICP* 1991;25:54–64.
A review of the physiology of neuromuscular transmission and pharmacology of common neuromuscular blocking agents.

Watling SM, Dasta JF. Prolonged paralysis in intensive care unit patients after the use of neuromuscular blocking agents: a review of the literature. *Crit Care Med* 1994;22:884–893.
A review of prolonged neuromuscular blockade caused by vecuronium and atracurium and proposed causes for this phenomenon based on case reports and studies in the literature.

NONSTEROIDAL ANTIINFLAMMATORY DRUGS

Ivan E. Liang

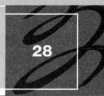

I. GENERAL PRINCIPLES

A. Nonsteroidal antiinflammatory drugs (NSAIDs) include aspirin, other salicylates, and a variety of other aspirinlike drugs. NSAIDs have analgesic, antipyretic, and antiinflammatory activity.

B. Therapeutic effects and gastrointestinal (GI) and renal side effects are caused by inhibition of cyclooxygenase and prostaglandin synthesis.

C. Aspirin is the only NSAID with significant antiplatelet activity.

II. PATHOPHYSIOLOGY

A. Salicylates

1. Absorption can continue for 24 hours after an acute overdose because of delayed dissolution of tablets or formation of gastric concretions.

2. Following single therapeutic doses, salicylate is metabolized in the liver to the inactive metabolites. The remaining 10% of the dose is excreted unchanged in the urine.

3. When serum concentrations exceed 20 mg/dL, the metabolism becomes saturated and elimination changes from first-order to zero-order kinetics and the half-life increases from about 2.5 hours to as long as 40 hours. Renal excretion of salicylate then becomes the most important route of elimination.

4. Following overdose, direct stimulation of the respiratory center in the medulla by toxic salicylate concentrations results in a respiratory alkalosis.

5. The accumulation of salicylate in cells causes uncoupling of mitochondrial oxidative phosphorylation, which leads to the characteristic increased anion gap metabolic acidosis.

B. NSAIDs

1. Nonsalicylate NSAIDs are rapidly absorbed following ingestion; they have small volumes of distribution and are highly protein bound.

2. In contrast to salicylates, the metabolism of most nonsalicylate NSAIDs is not saturable and elimination follows first-order kinetics.

III. CLINICAL PRESENTATION

A. Salicylates

1. Salicylate poisoning can occur with acute as well as chronic overdose.
2. Severity should be assessed by direct evaluation of acid-base status (Table 28-1) and clinical manifestations rather than by the serum salicylate level or the Done nomogram.
   a. Mild poisoning is defined by the presence of alkalemia (serum pH higher than 7.4) and alkaluria (urine pH less than 6). Signs and symptoms include nausea, vomiting, abdominal pain, diaphoresis, headache, tinnitus, and tachypnea.
   b. Moderate poisoning is defined by a normal or alkaline serum pH and aciduria (urine pH less than 6). Gastrointestinal (GI) tract and neurologic symptoms are more pronounced. Arterial blood gas and electrolyte analysis reveal combined respiratory alkalosis and metabolic acidosis with an increased anion gap.
   c. Severe poisoning is defined by the presence of acidemia and aciduria. Signs and symptoms include coma, seizures, respiratory depression, shock, or noncardiogenic pulmonary edema. Because of GI, renal, and insensible fluid losses, dehydration is invariably present and often underestimated.

B. Other NSAIDs

1. Metabolic acidosis, coma, seizures, hepatic dysfunction, hypotension, and cardiovascular collapse are relatively common after phenylbutazone overdose.
2. Other nonsalicylate NSAIDs rarely cause severe poisoning. Typical findings include nausea, vomiting, abdominal pain, headache, confusion, tinnitus, drowsiness, and hyperventilation. Symptoms usually last several hours.
3. Tonic–clonic seizures and muscle twitching have been reported after mefenamic acid overdose.

TABLE 28-1   **Severity of Salicylate Poisoning**

Grade	Plasma pH	Urine pH	Underlying metabolic abnormality
Mild	>7.4	>6.0	Respiratory alkalosis
Moderate	=7.4	<6.0	Combined respiratory alkalosis and metabolic acidosis
Severe	<7.4	<6.0	Metabolic acidosis with or without respiratory acidosis

Source: Irwin RS, Rippe JM. *Irwin and Rippe's Intensive Care Medicine,* 5th ed. Philadelphia: Lippincott Williams & Wilkins, 2003:1553.

IV. EVALUATION

A. Salicylates

1. Initial laboratory evaluation should include arterial blood gases, electrolytes, glucose, blood urea nitrogen (BUN), and creatinine levels, and urinalysis.

2. In patients with moderate to severe poisoning, further evaluation should include determinations of serum calcium, magnesium, and ketones; liver function tests; complete blood cell count (CBC); coagulation studies; and an electrocardiogram (ECG) and chest radiograph.

3. Because patients often confuse aspirin and acetaminophen, toxicology testing should be done for both substances.

4. Serial salicylate levels should be performed to assess for continued drug absorption and the efficacy of decontamination and elimination therapies.

B. Other NSAIDs

1. The diagnostic evaluation of patients with acute NSAID overdose is the same as for salicylates.

2. Evaluation of acid-base, electrolyte, and renal parameters is particularly important.

3. Additional ancillary testing is dictated by clinical severity.

V. MANAGEMENT

A. Salicylates

1. Resuscitative measures should be instituted as necessary. If endotracheal intubation and mechanical ventilation are instituted, hyperventilation is essential to prevent acidemia and the resultant increased tissue penetration of salicylic acid into the central nervous system (CNS).

2. Noncardiac pulmonary edema should be treated with intubation and positive end-expiratory pressure (PEEP) rather than diuretics.

3. Because CNS hypoglycemia can occur despite a normal serum glucose, obtain a finger-stick blood sugar or empirically treat with $D_{50}W$ in patients with altered mental status.

4. GI tract decontamination should be performed in all patients with intentional overdoses and in those with accidental ingestions of greater than 150 mg/kg. It may be effective for as long as 24 hours following overdose and in patients with spontaneous vomiting, because of delayed absorption and concretion formation.
a. Activated charcoal without cathartic—the preferred therapy—should be given to all patients.
b. Gastric lavage and endoscopy may have a role in patients with large ingestions and rising drug levels despite charcoal therapy.

5. The administration of multiple-dose charcoal may enhance salicylate elimination and should also be considered, but the clinical efficacy of this therapy is debatable.

6. Initial fluid therapy should be intravenous 5% dextrose in normal saline or 5% dextrose in one-half normal saline with one ampule (50 mEq) of

TABLE 28-2	Alkaline Diuresis Therapy of Salicylate Poisoning: Fluid and Electrolyte Therapy[a]		
Grade	**Intravenous solution**	**NaHCO₃ (amp/L)**	**Potassium (mEq/L)**
Mild	D_5NS	1	20
Moderate	$D_5^1/_2NS$	2	40
Severe	D_5W	3	60

Source: Irwin RS, Rippe JM. *Irwin and Rippe's Intensive Care Medicine,* 5th ed. Philadelphia: Lippincott Williams & Wilkins, 2003:1557.
D_5NS, 5% dextrose in normal saline; $D_5^1/_2NS$, 5% dextrose in one-half normal saline; D_5W, 5% dextrose in water; NaHCO₃, 50 mEq sodium bicarbonate/50 mL ampule (8.4%).
[a]Initial treatment should include hydration with 1–3 L of a saline solution containing dextrose (see text).

sodium bicarbonate and potassium (10 to 20 mEq/L) with 1 to 3 L given over the first 1 to 2 hours.

7. Electrolyte abnormalities should be corrected.
8. Salicylate elimination can be enhanced by urinary alkalinization and diuresis and extracorporeal removal.
   a. Indications for urinary alkalinization include systemic symptoms, acid-base abnormalities, or salicylate levels greater than 30 mg/dL after an acute overdose.
      (1) The goal is to achieve a urine pH of 7.5 or greater and a urine output of 2 to 4 mL/kg/h (Table 28-2).
      (2) Additional boluses of bicarbonate should be given to correct acidemia.
      (3) Acetazolamide should not be used to alkalinize the urine because it can cause a concomitant systemic acidosis, which may promote tissue distribution of salicylate and result in clinical deterioration.
      (4) Alkali therapy should be withheld if the serum pH is greater than 7.55.
   d. Hemodialysis is indicated in patients with severe poisoning and in those with moderate poisoning who fail to respond to alkaline diuresis.
      (1) It is generally necessary for patients with serum levels greater than 1,000 mg/L (100 mg/dL) after an acute intoxication and 600 mg/L (60 mg/dL) after chronic intoxication, but severe or progressive clinical toxicity is the most important indication.
      (2) It is essential for a successful outcome in those with coma, seizures, cerebral or pulmonary edema, or renal failure.

B. Other NSAIDs
1. The treatment of nonsalicylate NSAID poisoning is supportive and symptomatic.
2. Advanced life support measures and invasive monitoring may be required in severe cases.

3. Renal function should be monitored carefully in patients with abnormal urinalysis, underlying renal disease, or advanced age.

4. GI tract decontamination with activated charcoal is recommended for patients who present soon after ingestion (see Chapter 1).

Selected Readings

Balali-Mood M, Critchley JA, Proudfoot AT, et al. Mefenamic acid overdose. *Lancet* 1981;1354–1356.
A case series of mefenamic acid overdose that showed a high number of patients with neurologic toxicity, such as seizures and muscle twitching.

Brenner BE, Simon RR. Management of salicylate intoxication. *Drugs* 1982;24:335–340.
A review article on salicylate toxicity with a discussion of the different bedside tests for salicylates.

Duffens KR, Smilkstein MJ, Bessen HA, et al. Falsely elevated salicylate levels due to diflunisal overdose. *J Emerg Med* 1987;5:499–503.
A case report and discussion of the cross-reactivity of diflunisal with the immunoassay and colorimetric assay for salicylates.

Dugandzic RM, Tierney MG, Dickinson GE, et al. Evaluation of the validity of the Done nomogram in the management of acute salicylate intoxication. *Ann Emerg Med* 1989;18:1186–1190.
A retrospective study of 55 acute salicylate intoxications, which demonstrated that management decisions should be based on the clinical presentation and serum salicylate level.

Gabow PA, Anderson RJ, Potts DE, et al. Acid-base disturbances in the salicylate intoxicated adult. *Arch Intern Med* 1978;138:1481–1484.
A retrospective study of 67 adults with salicylate toxicity focusing on acid-base disturbances. The presence of acidemia in this group correlated with neurologic symptoms.

Hall AH, Smolinske SC, Conrad FL, et al. Ibuprofen overdose: 126 cases. *Ann Emerg Med* 1986;15:1308–1313.
A retrospective review of 126 ibuprofen overdose cases in adults and children. Ibuprofen toxicity in most cases was benign, but two children had seizures and one child died.

Hill JB. Experimental salicylate poisoning: observations on the effects of altering blood pH on tissue and plasma salicylate concentrations. *Pediatrics* 1971;47:658–665.
An experimental model that demonstrated the importance of serum pH on the distribution of salicylates. Acidemia facilitates salicylate distribution into the brain.

Johnson D, Eppler J, Giesbrecht E, et al. Effect of multiple-dose activated charcoal on the clearance of high-dose intravenous aspirin in a porcine model. *Ann Emerg Med* 1995;26:569–574.
An animal model showing no benefit of multiple-dose activated charcoal in the clearance of high-dose aspirin.

Linden CH, Townsend PL. Metabolic acidosis after acute ibuprofen overdosage. *J Pediatr* 1987;111;922–925.
Two case reports and a discussion of the increased anion gap after acute ibuprofen overdose.

McGuigan MA. A two-year review of salicylate deaths in Ontario. *Arch Intern Med* 1987;147:510–512.
A retrospective study of salicylate deaths that demonstrated specific management difficulties such as establishing the diagnosis, administering activated charcoal, and using hemodialysis.

Notarianni L. A reassessment of the treatment of salicylate poisoning. *Drug Saf* 1992;7: 292–303.
A review article focusing on the recent developments in salicylate toxicity, including the discouragement of forced diuresis to enhance elimination.

Smith MJH. The metabolic basis of the major symptoms in acute salicylate intoxication. *Clin Toxicol* 1968;1:387–407.
The classic paper on the effects of salicylates on metabolism and the clinical symptoms.

Smolinske SC, Hall AH, Vandenberg SA, et al. Toxic effects of nonsteroidal anti-inflammatory drugs in overdose: an overview of recent evidence on clinical effects and dose–response relationships. *Drug Saf* 1990;5:253–274.
The clinical effects and toxicity of 26 different nonsteroidal antiinflammatory drugs are discussed.

Veltri JC, Rollins DE. A comparison of the frequency and severity of poisoning cases for ingestion of acetaminophen, aspirin, and ibuprofen. *Am J Emerg Med* 1988;6: 104–107.
Data from the American Association of Poison Control Centers regarding exposure to analgesics revealed that the majority of patients had a low rate of serious effects.

Wortzman DJ, Grunfeld A. Delayed absorption following enteric-coated aspirin overdose. *Ann Emerg Med* 1987;16:434–436.
A case report of delayed toxicity following an overdose of sustained-release salicylate preparation.

I. BACKGROUND

A. Opioids are a diverse group of substances that have morphine-like analgesic effects.

B. Toxicity results from exaggerated pharmacologic activity.

II. PATHOPHYSIOLOGY

A. Opioids bind to and stimulate opioid receptors in the central nervous system (CNS).

  1. μ-Receptor stimulation leads to analgesia as well as sedation, euphoria, miosis, and constipation. Reduced sensitivity of medullary chemoreceptors to hypercarbia and hypoxia leads to respiratory depression.

  2. κ-Receptor stimulation produces analgesia, dysphoria, and psychotic features. Pentazocine binds to this receptor.

  3. σ-Receptor stimulation causes psychosis and movement disorders. Naloxone does not antagonize these effects. Both dextromethorphan and pentazocine bind at this receptor.

B. Downstream effects on dopamine are likely responsible for the myoclonic activity that can develop after administration of any opioid.

C. Opioids can directly cause mast cell degranulation and histamine release.

D. Most opiates are well absorbed from multiple routes of administration, including intravenous (IV), intramuscular (IM), subcutaneous (SC), inhalational, oral, and mucosal (sublingual, intranasal).

  1. Heat instability prevents smoking most agents except black tar heroin.

  2. Significant first-pass metabolism limits the oral bioavailability of most opioids.

E. Peak plasma concentrations generally occur within 1 to 2 hours after therapeutic oral dosing.

  1. Decreased gastrointestinal (GI) motility in overdose or coingestion with anticholinergics may prolong the absorption phase.

  2. Duration of action is prolonged after oral overdose, particularly with methadone and sustained-release formulations (e.g., MSContin, Oxycontin).

F. Opioids are metabolized by hepatic hydroxylation, demethylation, and glucoronide conjugation. Metabolites are eliminated through renal excretion.

III. DIAGNOSIS

A. Clinical Toxicity

1. Patients may become poisoned after accidental intravenous heroin overdose, intentional or accidental oral overdose, or therapeutic misadventures.

2. Regardless of the particular opioid or route of exposure, the classic opioid toxidrome consists of CNS and respiratory depression.

3. Miosis is common, with the exceptions of meperidine, propoxyphene, pentazocine, coingestion with anticholinergic or sympathomimetic drugs, and severe anoxic brain injury.

4. Variable effects include euphoria, dysphoria, nausea, decreased bowel activity, myoclonus, hypotension, pruritis, and pulmonary edema.

5. Noncardiogenic pulmonary edema is common with heroin overdose but may be seen with any opioid overdose. Hypoxemia, rales, and x-ray findings may be delayed several hours after overdose.

6. Considerations with respect to specific agents

   a. Heroin has two to five times the potency of morphine. Purity of street sources ranges from 5% to 90%. Adulterants such quinidine, strychnine, lidocaine, cocaine, and scopolamine used for cutting or bulking street heroin may cause additional toxicity. Track marks (scarred veins) or "skin popping" lesions (scarred skin and subcutaneous tissue) may be seen in injection users.

   b. Fentanyl has a potency 200 times that of morphine. Transdermal patches are sometimes intentionally ingested or smoked. Rapid IV boluses can produce profound truncal rigidity, impairing ventilation. More potent derivatives, such as alpha-methyl-fentanyl (China White), are produced in clandestine laboratories and sold as heroin substitutes.

   c. Meperidine has a propensity to cause dysphoria and hallucinations. Other unique effects include CNS excitation, tremors, muscle twitching, mydriasis, and seizures. Seizures can result from accumulation of the normeperidine metabolite, which occurs with high IV doses, repeated oral dosing (first-pass hepatic metabolism) and renal failure (decreased metabolite excretion).

   d. Diphenoxylate with atropine (Lomotil) decreases GI motility and is used for diarrhea. One tablet can produce serious toxicity in a child; 1.2 mg/kg is potentially fatal. Onset of toxicity can be delayed up to 30 hours. The atropine component can cause anticholinergic poisoning (see Chapter 5).

   e. Methadone is a long-acting opioid used primarily for detoxification or maintenance therapy in opioid addicts. As little as 40 mg can cause coma in nontolerant individuals. Prolonged effects can be expected.

   f. Propoxyphene is notable for its ability to cause cardiac toxicity and seizures. Cardiovascular effects include hypotension, QRS widening, and ventricular tachycardia and are the result of the sodium channel blocking effects (see Chapter 4) of the drug and its norpropoxyphene metabolite.

   g. Pentazocine has both agonist and antagonist activity at opioid receptors. Anxiety and dysphoria are common.

h. Dextromethorphan lacks analgesic and euphoric effects at therapeutic doses and is used as an antitussive. Large doses can cause increased perceptual awareness, altered time perception, and visual hallucinations. It is commonly abused by teenagers. Medications containing this opioid may also contain antihistamines or decongestants, which can also cause anticholinergic and sympathomimetic toxicity, respectively (see Chapters 5 and 33). Long-term abuse can lead to bromism (mental confusion, stupor, delusions, headache, hallucinations, nervousness, and weakness) because the drug is formulated as a bromide salt.

i. Tramadol has only moderate affinity for the μ-receptor. Analgesic effects likely stem from its ability to block the reuptake of biogenic amines in descending neural pathways. Adverse effects include seizures (as may occur in therapeutic dosing) and serotonin syndrome (see Chapter 7).

7. Histamine release can result in local or generalized flushing and itching, sometimes with hypotension. Red streaks may be noted along the course of a vein used for injection.

B. Evaluation

1. Cardiac and oxygen saturation monitoring should be performed in symptomatic patients and those with acute overdose.

2. A chest radiograph, electrocardiogram (ECG), and routine laboratory studies are indicated in patients with coma, hypotension, abnormal cardiac rhythm, hypoxemia, or abnormal cardiopulmonary examination.

3. Packets of heroin may be seen on plain radiograph in the case of "body packers" or "body stuffers" (see Chapter 14). Addition of gastrograffin or use of a computed tomography (CT) scan may aid in the diagnosis if plain films are unrevealing.

4. Urine drugs of abuse immunoassays often use antibodies to morphine and can detect only this drug and its congeners heroin (diacetylmorphine) and codeine (methylmorphine). Semisynthetic opioids such as oxycodone and synthetic agents such as fentanyl generally are not detected.

a. Clinicians should ask about the sensitivity of the assay used.

b. The diagnosis is clinical, however, making urine assays superfluous.

c. Serum concentrations are not clinically useful.

IV. TREATMENT

A. Oxygen and bag-valve mask ventilation are critical initial interventions in apneic or severely bradypneic patients.

B. Naloxone, a rapid-acting μ-receptor antagonist, should then be administered.

1. It can be given IV, IM, SC, or via endotracheal tube but is ineffective when given orally.

2. The goal of therapy is to restore adequate spontaneous ventilation.

3. Using naloxone to achieve complete arousal may precipitate opioid withdrawal in tolerant patients.

4. Accidental overdose in opioid abusers or tolerant individuals generally responds to low doses (0.05 mg to 0.1 mg IV), whereas intentional overdose, and particularly ingestions by nontolerant individuals, may require large doses (up to 10 mg). An initial dose of 0.4 to 2.0 mg IV is recommended in the latter situation.

5. If toxic effects persist or recur, incremental or repeated doses should be given.

6. Alternatively, a naloxone infusion may be given for recurrent toxicity (e.g., for methadone, sustained-release formulation, body packers).

   a. Begin with an hourly rate equal to two-thirds the bolus dose needed to reverse toxicity.

   b. Increase or decrease the rate of infusion by 50% as needed to prevent respiratory depression or withdrawal, respectively.

C. Intubation is indicated for CNS and respiratory depression if naloxone is unavailable, delayed, or ineffective.

D. Seizures should be treated with naloxone and benzodiazepines.

E. Hypotension should be treated with IV saline and dopamine.

F. QRS widening and ventricular tachycardia resulting from propoxyphene overdose should be treated with sodium bicarbonate and lidocaine (see Chapter 4).

G. Activated charcoal should be considered for recent oral overdoses (see Chapter 1).

H. Whole bowel irrigation and activated charcoal (see Chapter 1) should be considered for body packers and body stuffers. Surgical removal may be necessary for intestinal perforation or obstruction.

I. Disposition

1. Accidental heroin overdose

   a. Patients who remain asymptomatic and have normal oxygen saturation after treatment with naloxone can be discharged after being observed for 2 to 4 hours.

   b. Those who remain symptomatic or hypoxemic after naloxone should be admitted to a location capable of continuous monitoring of oxygen saturation and ventilation.

2. Oral opioid overdose

   a. Patients with intentional overdose and children with accidental ingestion require prolonged (12- to 24-hour) observation because of the potential for delayed absorption and toxicity.

   b. Admission to a unit capable of continuous monitoring of oxygen saturation and ventilation is recommended.

V. COMPLICATIONS

A. Complications include aspiration, pulmonary edema, rhabdomyolysis, and anoxic brain injury.

B. Additional complications may result from adulterant and coingestant effects.

Selected Reading

Goldfrank K, Weisman RS, Errick JK, et al. A dosing nomogram for continuous infusion intravenous naloxone. *Ann Emerg Med* 1986;15:566–570.
This study determined an appropriate dosing protocol for naloxone infusion.

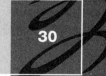
I. BACKGROUND

A. In addition to organophosphorous and carbamate compounds (see Chapter 13), agents used as pesticides include aluminum and zinc phosphide, anticoagulants, DEET (N,N-diethyl-m-toluamide), methyl bromide, organochlorine compounds, paraquat and diquat, sodium monofluoroacetate (SMFA, Compound 1080), and strychnine.

B. Each of these unrelated agents has a unique mechanism of action and therapy.

C. Regardless of the agent involved, management of exposure involves limiting chemical absorption, protection of rescue personnel, and supportive measures.

1. Remove clothing and wash the skin with soap and water to eliminate residue following topical exposures.

2. Perform decontamination in a well-vented area.

3. Use of chemical-resistant gowns, nitrile gloves, shoe covers, and eye protection may be appropriate.

II. PATHOPHYSIOLOGY

A. Aluminum and Zinc Phosphide

1. Used as fumigant and grain preservative.

2. Phosphine, a corrosive gas that smells like decaying fish and inhibits cytochrome oxidase, is released when phosphides react with moisture.

3. Poisoning may result from ingestion of phosphides or inhalation of phosphine.

B. Anticoagulants

1. Used as a rodenticide in bait form.

2. Include warfarin and the "superwarfarin" agents (brodifacoum, difenacoum, and indanedione derivatives).

3. Superwarfarins are approximately 100 times more potent than warfarin and have a much longer half-life.

4. Inhibit vitamin K 2,3-epoxide reductase and vitamin K reductase, which are responsible for the regeneration of vitamin K, a coenzyme responsible for activation of clotting factors II, VII, IX, and X as well as anticoagulant proteins C and S.

C. DEET

1. Active ingredient in topical insect repellents.
2. Causes neurotoxicity, but mechanism of action is unknown.
3. Poisoning may result from the skin application of concentrated DEET preparations, repeated application of diluted formulations, or ingestion.

D. Methyl Bromide

1. Colorless gas used as a fumigant to control for nematodes, insects, rodents, fungi, and weeds.
2. Appears to act by methylating sulfhydryl groups on intracellular enzymes.

E. Organochlorines

1. Used topically as insecticides, soil fumigants, and herbicides.
2. Examples include endrin, dieldrin, aldrin, chlordane, dichlorodiphenyl trichloroethane (DDT), and lindane (Kwell).
3. Systemic toxicity can occur by ingestion, dermal absorption, or inhalation.

F. Paraquat and Diquat

1. Structurally similar and used as topical herbicides and defoliants.
2. Free radical metabolites react with oxygen to form superoxide radicals, which then cause lipid peroxidation and cellular destruction.
3. Paraquat is selectively taken up by alveolar cells of the lung.

G. SMFA

1. Used primarily in bait to exterminate rodents and larger mammals.
2. Fluoroacetate enters the tricarboxylic acid cycle where it is metabolized to fluorocitrate, which disrupts the cycle and halts cellular respiration.

H. Strychnine

1. Used in animal bait and, rarely, as an adulterant in illicit drugs.
2. Competitively antagonizes inhibitory postsynaptic glycine receptors in the spinal cord, resulting in neuromuscular disinhibition and contraction of both flexor and extensor muscle groups.

III. DIAGNOSIS

A. Clinical Toxicity

1. Aluminum and zinc phosphide
   a. Inhalation of phosphine results in eye and throat irritation, cough, dyspnea, pulmonary edema, cardiovascular depression, conduction disturbances, and arrhythmias.
   b. Ingestion of phosphides initially causes nausea, vomiting, and abdominal pain. Respiratory symptoms can be delayed several hours.
2. Anticoagulants
   a. Anticoagulant effects include spontaneous cutaneous bleeding, soft-tissue ecchymosis, gingival bleeding, epistaxis, and hematuria.
   b. Onset may be delayed for 24 hours or more after ingestion.

3. DEET

    a. Anaphylactic reactions have been reported with cutaneous application.

    b. Systemic effects include anxiety, behavioral changes, tremors, lethargy, ataxia, confusion, seizures, and coma.

4. Methyl bromide

    a. Symptoms can be delayed 6 hours or longer after exposure.

    b. Manifestations of mild poisoning include dizziness, headache, confusion, weakness, nausea, vomiting, and dyspnea.

    c. Skin irritation and burns can occur under clothes and rubber gloves where gas is trapped.

    d. Severe poisoning can result in tremor, myoclonus, pulmonary edema, seizures, and coma.

5. Organochlorines

    a. Cause seizures as well as central nervous system (CNS) depression.

    b. Seizures may occur without a prodrome.

    c. Eldrin can cause hyperthermia and decerebrate posturing.

    d. Ingestion may result in vomiting and diarrhea.

    e. Cardiac dysrhythmias have been reported.

6. Paraquat and diquat

    a. Ingestion of more than 40 mg/kg of paraquat can be fatal.

    b. Initial toxicity includes corrosive esophagitis and gastrointestinal (GI) hemorrhage.

    c. Patients usually die within hours to days from multiple-organ failure including acute respiratory distress syndrome (ARDS), cerebral edema, myocardial necrosis, and hepatic and renal failure.

    d. Patients who ingest 20 to 40 mg/kg of paraquat may die from pulmonary fibrosis, which progresses over a period of days to weeks.

    e. Similar toxicity is seen with diquat, but diquat does not affect the pulmonary system.

7. SMFA

    a. Initial symptoms are nausea and vomiting.

    b. Later symptoms are agitation, seizures, coma, ventricular arrhythmias, and hypotension.

    c. Metabolic acidosis and hypocalcemia with QT interval prolongation can occur.

8. Strychnine

    a. Onset of toxicity is rapid, usually within 15 to 30 minutes.

    b. Facial muscle spasm results in risus sardonicus ("sardonic smile") and trismus.

    c. Opisthotonos and muscle contractions and convulsions resemble seizures and can lead to respiratory failure, but mental status remains clear.

    d. Effects usually resolve within 12 to 24 hours.

B. Evaluation

1. Laboratory studies in symptomatic patients should include routine serum chemistries.

2. Coagulation studies are appropriate for those with anticoagulant exposures.

3. A chest x-ray and electrocardiogram should be obtained in patients with cardiovascular or respiratory complaints or findings.

4. Serum bromide levels may be elevated in methyl bromide poisoning but are not helpful in determining the severity of exposure.

5. Serum paraquat levels correlate with toxicity but are not readily available.

IV. TREATMENT

A. Advanced life support measures should be instituted as necessary.

B. Seizures should be treated with benzodiazepines and barbiturates.

   1. Benzodiazepines and barbiturates are the agents of choice in terminating strychnine-induced muscle contractions.

   2. Nondepolarizing muscle blockers may be required for refractory convulsions.

C. Multiple-dose activated charcoal (see Chapter 1) should be considered for patients with organochlorine and paraquat/diquat ingestions.

D. Magnesium may be useful for arrhythmias caused by phosphides, phosphine, or SMFA.

E. Hypocalcemia and prolonged QT interval resulting from SMFA overdose should be treated with intravenous calcium.

F. Vitamin K_1 (phytonadione) is the only form of vitamin K that is effective for treatment of coagulopathy resulting from anticoagulant poisoning.

   1. It can be given orally, subcutaneously, intramuscularly, or intravenously.

   2. Treatment duration is highly variable and must be titrated to clinical and laboratory response.

   3. Fresh frozen plasma should be reserved for life-threatening bleeding.

G. Hemoperfusion may be helpful in enhancing the elimination of paraquat if performed soon after ingestion.

H. Measures that may decrease pulmonary toxicity from paraquat include limiting oxygen therapy to that which is absolutely necessary and immunosuppressive therapy with cyclophosphamide (15 mg/kg/day for 2 days), methylprednisolone (15 mg/kg/day for 6 days), and dexamethasone (5 mg every 8 hours).

Selected Readings

Cohn WJ, Boylan JJ, Blanke RV, et al. Treatment of chlordecone (Kepone) toxicity with cholestyramine. *N Engl J Med* 1978;298:243–248.
   A clinical study demonstrating increased elimination of chlordecone with administration of cholestyramine.

Edmunds M, Sheehan TM, Van't Hoff W. Strychnine poisoning: clinical and toxicological observations on a non-fatal case. *J Toxicol Clin Toxicol* 1986;24:245–255.
   A case report and general discussion of strychnine poisoning and its management.

Egekeze JO, Oehme FW. Sodium monofluoroacetate (SMFA, compound 1080): a literature review. *Vet Hum Toxicol* 1979;21:411–416.
   A review of sodium monofluoroacetate describing the pathophysiology, toxicity, and treatment.

Hart RB, Nevitt A, Whitehead A. A new statistical approach to the prognostic significance of plasma paraquat concentrations. *Lancet* 1984;2:1222–1223.
An analysis of 219 paraquat-poisoned patients that constructs survival based on serum paraquat concentration and time since ingestion.

Hine CH. Methyl bromide poisoning: a review of ten cases. *J Occup Med* 1969; 11:1–10.
A case series of patients describing sources and clinical toxicity of methyl bromide.

Katona B, Wason S. Superwarfarin poisoning. *J Emerg Med* 1989;7:627–631.
A review article describing clinical toxicity of superwarfarin compounds, including a suggested approach to the management of patients with intentional and unintentional rodenticide ingestions.

Pond SM. Manifestations and management of paraquat poisoning. *Med J Aust* 1990; 152:256–259.
An excellent review of the pathophysiology, clinical toxicity, and management of paraquat poisoning.

Seizures temporally associated with use of DEET insect repellent—New York and Connecticut. *MMWR* 1989;38:678–680.
A report of seizures after cutaneous exposure to DEET.

Wilson R, Lovejoy FH, Jaeger RJ, et al. Acute phosphine poisoning aboard a grain freighter: epidemiologic, clinical, and pathological findings. *JAMA* 1980;244: 148–150.
A case series of patients who developed acute phosphine poisoning; contains a description of the clinical presentation and epidemiology of these poisonings.

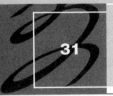

PHENCYCLIDINE AND HALLUCINOGENS
D. Eric Brush

I. BACKGROUND

A. Phencyclidine (PCP) is a dissociative anesthetic that is structurally similar to ketamine, which causes out-of-body experiences as well as central nervous system (CNS) stimulation or depression.

   1. PCP is available as an acid (white crystalline powder) or in alkaloid (grayish-white) form. Both may be injected or ingested. The alkaloid is sometimes incorporated into marijuana and smoked.

   2. Ketamine, along with multiple PCP analogs, is frequently sold as a PCP substitute.

B. Hallucinogens are analogs of amphetamine (phenylethylamines) or tryptamine (indolamines), which cause "tripping" (auditory and visual hallucinations) along with variable degrees of CNS stimulation.

   1. Lysergic acid diethylamide (LSD) is sold as squares of dipped blotter paper, microdots (dried residue), liquid, and gelatin squares. Other lysergamides are found in morning glory seeds (*Rivea* and *Ipomoea* sp.). Several hundred seeds are required for hallucinogenic effects.

   2. Psilocybin and psilocin are found in *Psilocybe* and other hallucinogenic mushrooms ("magic mushrooms"), which are dried and sold whole or in powdered form.

   3. N,N-dimethyltryptamine (DMT) from the Yakee plant (*Virola calophylla*) is available as a liquid or yellow-tan powder.

   4. 5-methoxy-N,N-dimethyltryptamine (5-MeO-DMT) is sold as white crystals. It is also found in the secretions of the *Bufo* sp. toads (along with bufotenine–5-hydroxydimethyltryptamine).

   5. Dimethoxymethylamphetamine (DOM), methylenedioxyamphetamine (MDA), p-methoxyamphetamine (PMA), methylenedioxymethamphetamine (MDMA, "ecstacy" or "XTC"), and methylenedioxyethamphetamine (MDEA, "eve") are available as tablets, powders, or "window panes" (gelatin squares).

   6. Dextromethorphan (DXM) is found in a variety of cold remedies, often combined with antihistamines or decongestants.

   7. Mescaline is the active agent in the peyote cactus (*Lophophora williamsii*). The "button" of the cactus is ingested.

C. Anticholinergic compounds (e.g., belladonna alkaloids in the seeds of jimson weed or *Datura stramonium*) are also hallucinogenic (see Chapter 5).

II. PATHOPHYSIOLOGY

A. Phencyclidine and Ketamine

1. These agents have multiple actions, including N-methyl-D-aspartate (NMDA) receptor antagonism, biogenic amine reuptake blockade, serotonin antagonism, and at very high doses nicotinic, muscarinic, and opiate receptor activity.
2. They are readily absorbed by all routes, have large volumes of distribution and high protein binding, and are hepatically metabolized.
3. Onset of action is rapid. PCP effects may last 6 to 24 hours, and some alterations in perception persist up to 3 days. The duration of effect of ketamine depends on the route of administration (intravenously [IV], 15 min; intramuscularly [IM], 30 to 120 min; nasally, 45 to 90 min., by mouth [PO], 4 to 8 h).

B. Hallucinogens

1. These agents act by modulating serotonin neurotransmission. Amphetamine derivatives also have sympathomimetic effects.
2. All are well absorbed from the gastrointestinal (GI) route, with the notable exceptions of DMT and 5-MeO-DMT, which are degraded by intestinal monoamine oxidase enzymes. Metabolism is hepatic.
3. Effects usually begin in 30 to 60 minutes, but duration of action varies: up to 12 hours for LSD and mescaline, 4 to 6 hours for *Psilocybe* mushrooms, and 12 to 36 hours for 4-bromo-2,5-dimethoxyamphetamine (DOB).
4. DMT and 5-MeO-DMT have rapid onset (minutes) and short duration of action (1 hour).

III. DIAGNOSIS

A. Clinical Toxicity

1. PCP and ketamine cause dissociation from reality and inability to interpret external stimuli, leading to decreased pain sensation and difficulty comprehending reality.
   a. This may lead to feelings of invincibility, resulting in trauma.
   b. Patients may appear intoxicated, agitated, lethargic, calm, mute, or comatose. The level of consciousness may fluctuate.
   c. Behavior may be violent and unpredictable. Some individuals may display extraordinary strength, making restraint difficult.
   d. Visual or auditory hallucinations occur in about 20% of patients.
   e. Vital signs may reveal hyperthermia, labile hypertension, or tachycardia.
   f. Multidirectional nystagmus (horizontal, vertical, and rotatory) is a pathognomonic finding.
   g. Rigidity of extremities, oculogyric crisis, trismus, facial grimacing, circumoral muscle twitching, lip smacking, torticollis, tongue spasms, opisthotonus, cataplexy, hyperreflexia, and clonus may be present.
   h. Neuromuscular hyperactivity commonly results in rhabdomyolysis.

2. Hallucinogen users rarely present to medical care unless they experience a "bad trip" (the inability to separate hallucinations from reality leads to uncontrolled panic) or trauma.
   a. Symptoms include auditory and visual hallucinations, distorted time perception, and delusions.
   b. Hallucinogen persisting perceptual disorder (flashbacks) may occur with LSD, morning glory seeds, or *Psilocybe* mushrooms and be precipitated by stress, illness, or exercise.
   c. Hypertension, tachycardia, and hyperthermia may be present.
   d. Rhabdomyolysis can occur.
   e. Patients who dance for prolonged periods at a "rave" party may drink large quantities of hypotonic fluids and present with lethargy and weakness owing to hyponatremia.

B. **Differential Diagnosis.** Other causes of altered mental status, such as hypoglycemia, CNS pathology (infection, bleeding, tumor), alcohol or sedative-hypnotic withdrawal, and psychiatric disease, should be considered.

C. **Evaluation**
   1. Laboratory evaluation should include bedside glucose to rule out hypoglycemia, complete blood count (CBC), routine serum chemistries, and creatine phosphokinase (CPK).
   2. Immunoassays do not detect most hallucinogens, with the exception of PCP. Dextromethorphan can cause a false-positive PCP screen.

IV. TREATMENT

A. Advanced life support measures should be instituted as necessary.
B. Most patients do well with minimal stimulation, such as in a dark, quiet room.
C. Violent patients may require physical and chemical restraints to prevent self-harm or staff injury.
   1. Benzodiazepines should be used liberally to control neuromuscular hyperactivity.
   2. Haloperidol and chlorpromazine may also be useful for PCP intoxication.
D. Cooling measures are typically not needed for mild hyperthermia if the patient is well sedated; however, failure to respond to sedation or the presence of profound hyperthermia (107°F) warrants more aggressive treatment, such as intubation, chemical paralysis, and active cooling measures.
E. IV fluids are recommended to treat rhabdomyolysis.
F. Activated charcoal (see Chapter 1) is unlikely to be helpful but should be considered for recent ingestions (e.g., multiple morning glory seeds).
G. Hyponatremia from water intoxication should be treated with fluid restriction.
H. Agitated delirium from anticholinergic poisoning may be reversed with physostigmine (see Chapter 5).

V. COMPLICATIONS

A. Complications include associated trauma, aspiration, rhabdomyolysis, hyponatremia, and multiple-organ failure from hyperthermia.

B. Most patients can be discharged to a responsible party after they are calm and oriented and such complications have been excluded.

Selected Readings

Burns RS, Lerner SE. Perspectives: acute phencyclidine intoxication. *Clin Toxicol* 1976;9:477–501.
An extensive discussion about the acute effects of phencyclidine toxicity.

Callaway CW, Clark RF. Hyperthermia in psychostimulant overdose. *Ann Emerg Med* 1994;24:68–76.
An excellent review article about the current understanding of the treatment of hyperthermia in overdose patients.

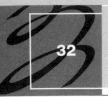

SEDATIVE-HYPNOTICS
D. Eric Brush

I. BACKGROUND

    A. Sedative-hypnotic agents are a chemically diverse group of drugs with the common feature of causing general central nervous system (CNS) depression.

    B. They are used to treat a wide variety of conditions, such as anxiety, insomnia, musculoskeletal disorders, seizures, and withdrawal states, and for anesthesia.

    C. The major drug classes are benzodiazepines (BZDs), barbiturates, and miscellaneous nonbenzodiazepine–nonbarbiturate sedative-hypnotics (Table 32-1).

    D. Acute intoxication leads to generalized CNS depression. Respiratory depression is variable depending on the agent. Other effects include hypotension and myocardial depression.

    E. Tolerance develops with chronic administration. Cross-tolerance may also occur between different sedatives. Withdrawal symptoms, including agitation, anxiety, hypertension, and seizures, may develop with abstinence after chronic use (see Chapter 35).

II. PATHOPHYSIOLOGY

A. Pharmacology

    1. BZDs bind to BZD receptors (omega 1, 2, or 3) in the CNS. This receptor is part of the γ-aminobutyric acid-A (GABA-A) receptor complex. Binding facilitates GABA neurotransmission by increasing the frequency of Cl^- ion influx through the receptor channel, causing net CNS depression.

    2. Barbiturates bind to the GABA-A receptor complex, causing the ion channel to remain open longer and thereby facilitating Cl^- flux and GABA-mediated CNS depression.

    3. Nonbenzodiazepine–nonbarbiturate agents are chemically distinct and diverse but pharmacologically similar. Many act through facilitation of GABA-A neurotransmission (chloral hydrate, meprobamate, methaqualone, zolpidem, γ-hydroxybutyrate acid [GHB]). Baclofen is a GABA-B agonist. GBH binds to GHB receptors associated with the GABA complex as well as to GABA-B receptors. Buspirone has serotonergic and dopaminergic as well as GABAergic activity.

B. Pharmacokinetics

    1. Gastrointestinal (GI) absorption of most agents is rapid. Exceptions are glutethimide, which has erratic absorption; meprobamate and

TABLE 32-1	Sedative-Hypnotic Agents Available in the United States

Benzodiazepines	Miscellaneous
Alprazolam	Alpidem[a]
Bromazepam[a]	Baclofen
Brotizolam[a]	Buspirone
Chlordiazepoxide	Chloral hydrate
Clobazam[a]	Chlormethiazole[a]
Clorazepate	Ethinamate
Diazepam	Ethchlorvynol
Estazolam	Glutethimide
Flunitrazepam	Meprobamate
Flurazepam	Methaqualone
Halazepam	Methyprylon
Lorazepam	Paraldehyde
Midazolam	Zolpidem
Nitrazepam	
Oxazepam	
Quazepam	
Triazolam	
Barbiturates	
Amobarbital	
Aprobarbital	
Butalbital	
Mephobarbital	
Pentobarbital	
Phenobarbital	
Secobarbital	
Thiopental	

Source: Irwin RS, Rippe JM. *Irwin and Rippe's Intensive Care Medicine,* 5th ed. Philadelphia: Lippincott Williams & Wilkins, 2003:1596.
[a]Investigational in the United States.

carisoprodol, which may form bezoars; and sustained-release mepro-bamate.

2. The onset and duration of clinical effects are partly determined by lipophilicity. More lipophilic drugs rapidly partition into the CNS gray matter and then redistribute to other tissues, leading to a rapid onset and brief duration of action. Other factors include a prolonged elimination phase and active metabolites (many BZDs, chloral hydrate).

3. Most sedatives are metabolized via the hepatic CYP-450 enzyme system. Exceptions include chloral hydrate (alcohol dehydrogenase metabolism), baclofen (mostly renal elimination), and GHB (precursor 1,4-BD is metabolized by alcohol dehydrogenase to GHB, which is metabolized via succinate semialdehyde).

4. Protein binding is extensive for most drugs in the class with the exception of chloral hydrate, meprobamate, and the longer-acting barbiturates (phenobarbital).

III. DIAGNOSIS

A. Clinical Manifestations of Overdose and Poisoning

1. Features common to all agents include ataxia, nystagmus, slurred speech, and CNS depression ranging from lethargy to coma. With deep coma, depression of respiratory, cardiovascular, and thermoregulatory centers in the brainstem can lead to apnea, hypotension, myocardial depression, hypothermia, and shock with cardiogenic or noncardiogenic pulmonary edema.

2. Unique findings include:

   a. BZDs: Deep coma is unusual and occurs only with massive overdose of short-acting agents such as temazepam and triazolam or when coingested with alcohol or other CNS depressants. Paradoxical agitation and anxiety may occur.

   b. Barbiturates: Coma can be rapid in onset (particularly with short-acting agents such as amobarbital, butalbital/butabarbital, pentobarbital, and secobarbital), prolonged (particularly with phenobarbital), and profound. Bullous skin lesions over pressure points and rhabdomyolysis can occur with prolonged coma.

   c. Chloral hydrate: Was added to ethanol in the "Mickey Finn." Lethal adult dose is 5 to 10 g, but significant toxicity may occur with doses as little as 1.25 g. Symptoms include GI irritation with nausea and vomiting and cardiac dysrhythmias, including ventricular tachycardia resulting from myocardial sensitization to endogenous catecholamines. Chloral hydrate may be seen as radiopaque material in the GI tract on plain film of the abdomen.

   d. Ethchlorvynol: Similar to phenobarbital. Half-life is prolonged, with overdose leading to prolonged coma. The aromatic (new plastic shower curtain) odor of the compound may be detected on the patient's breath.

   e. Glutethimide: Similar to phenobarbital. Active metabolite, which has a long duration of action and is more potent than the parent drug, leads to prolonged coma. Fluctuating level of consciousness (resulting from erratic absorption, redistribution from adipose tissue) and anticholinergic symptoms (see Chapter 5) may be seen.

   f. Methyprylon: Similar to phenobarbital. Adverse effects include nausea, vomiting, GI irritation, headache, rash, diarrhea, esophagitis, neutropenia, and thrombocytopenia.

   g. Meprobamate and carisoprodol: Meprobamate is a metabolite of carisoprodol. Toxicity of both is similar to that of glutethimide. Prolonged and erratic absorption (owing to bezoars and sustained-release preparations) can result in fluctuating level of consciousness.

   h. Baclofen: GABA-B agonism produces a distinct toxicity that includes hypertension (or hypotension), bradycardia (or tachycardia), hyperreflexia, myoclonus, and seizures as well as deep coma.

   i. Buspirone: Similar to BZDs, but experience is limited. Serotonin syndrome (see Chapter 7) can occur when administered with other serotonergic agents.

   j. Zolpidem and zaleplon. Similar to BZDs.

k. GHB: Similar to baclofen but with rapid onset (minutes) and short duration (several hours). Can produce euphoria and hallucinations as well as coma. Most users take a precursor drug (1,4-butanediol), which is converted by alcohol dehydrogenase to GHB. Coingestion with ethanol, which competes for metabolism, may delay toxicity. Another precursor, γ-butyrolactone, does not require enzymatic conversion.

B. Differential Diagnosis. Other causes of CNS depression include hypoglycemia, CNS infection, hemorrhage, or tumor and toxicity from ethanol, anticonvulsants, antidepressants, antihistamines, antipsychotics, and opiates.

C. Evaluation
1. Vital signs should include a rectal temperature in patients with coma because hypothermia may be overlooked.
2. Patients with coma should also have arterial blood gas analysis, complete blood count (CBC), electrolytes, blood urea nitrogen (BUN), creatinine, glucose, creatine phosphokinase (CPK; looking for possible rhabdomyolysis), electrocardiogram (ECG), and chest x-ray.
3. Check salicylate and acetaminophen concentrations, particularly with Fioricet and Fiorinal ingestions, which contain acetaminophen and aspirin respectively, as well as butalbital. Carisoprodol is also formulated with aspirin (Soma compound).
4. Urine drugs of abuse (immunoassay) screens detect most barbiturates, a minority of BZDs, and no other sedative-hypnotics.
5. Quantitative serum levels are not routinely available or clinically useful except for phenobarbital (therapeutic level 10 to 40 µg/mL) and perhaps other barbiturates.

IV. TREATMENT

A. Advanced life support measures should be instituted as necessary (see Chapter 1). Particular attention should be paid to protecting the airway and assisting ventilation via endotracheal intubation in patients with coma.
B. All patients should initially have continuous pulse-oximetry and cardiac monitoring along with IV access.
C. GI decontamination with activated charcoal should be considered for recent ingestions along with whole bowel irrigation for sustained-release meprobamate overdose (see Chapter 1).
D. Hypotension should initially be treated with several liters of IV saline. Vasopressors (e.g., dopamine, norepinephrine) should be used for refractory hypotension.
E. Ventricular tachyarrhythmias from chloral hydrate should be treated with β-blockers, lidocaine, and BZDs, as for other chlorinated hydrocarbons (see Chapter 20).
F. Bradydysrhythmias should be treated according to advanced cardiac life support (ACLS) guidelines, but epinephrine should be avoided in chloral hydrate poisoning (unless the patient is pulseless).

G. Seizures from baclofen or GHB can be treated with BZDs if prolonged or recurrent.

H. Rewarming measures should be instituted as needed for hypothermia.

I. IV flumazenil, a competitive inhibitor of BZD at central BZD receptors, can reverse CNS depression resulting from BZD, zolpidem, and zaleplon.

    1. For oral BZD overdose, the recommended dose is 0.2 mg, followed by 0.3 mg, then 0.5 mg doses to a maximum of 3 mg, each dose administered over 30 seconds and waiting 30 seconds for a response before giving the next dose. For partial responders, an additional 2 mg can be administered in increments of 0.5 mg.

    2. Since flumazenil can precipitate BZD withdrawal, an initial dose of 0.1 mg is prudent if chronic BZD use or tolerance is suspected.

    3. Relative contraindications include conditions for which BZDs may be therapeutic (e.g., coingestion of agents known to cause seizures, epilepsy).

    4. For reversal of BZD-induced procedural sedation, initial and subsequent doses of 0.2 mg (0.01 mg/kg, up to 0.2 mg per dose in children), up to a maximum of 1 mg, are recommended.

    5. Because abrupt reversal of BZD sedation can cause seizures in the absence of tolerance, administering doses slower than recommended (i.e., over 1 minute) may also be prudent.

J. Multidose activated charcoal and alkaline diuresis (see Chapter 1) can enhance the elimination of phenobarbital.

K. Hemodialysis can enhance the elimination of some agents and should be considered in patients with cardiovascular instability resulting from barbiturates, chloral hydrate, and meprobamate/carisoprodol who fail to respond to other measures. A rebound in blood levels may occur after hemodialysis as a result of drug redistribution.

V. COMPLICATIONS

A. Most patients do well with aggressive supportive care.

B. Complications include pressure-induced blisters, sores, and rhabdomyolysis, pulmonary edema, and anoxia- or shock-induced multiple-organ dysfunction.

Selected Readings

Berg MJ, Berlinger WG, Goldberg MJ, et al. Acceleration of the body clearance of phenobarbital by oral activated charcoal. *N Engl J Med* 1982;307:642–644.
Demonstrates the utility of activated charcoal for "gut dialysis" in the enhancement of phenobarbital clearance.

Spivey WH. Flumazenil and seizures: analysis of 43 cases. *Clin Ther* 1992;14:292–305.
This review of flumazenil-induced seizures highlights the need for cautious use in the reversal of BZD overdose, particularly in patients who coingest agents known to cause seizures or patients who have BZD tolerance.

I. BACKGROUND

A. Sympathomimetic agents include amphetamine (β-phenylisopropylamine) and its analogs (phenylethylamine family) such as methamphetamine, methylphenidate, dextroamphetamine, pemoline, and phentermine, which are used for treatment of attention deficit hyperactivity disorder (ADHD), narcolepsy, and weight reduction.

B. Clonidine (see Chapter 8) and related imidazolines, decongestants (oxymetaxoline, tetrahydrozoline), cocaine (see Chapter 14), ergot derivatives, hallucinogens (see Chapter 31), methylxanthines (see Chapter 26), monoamine oxidase inhibitors (see Chapter 7), and compounds found in over-the-counter cough and cold remedies, illicit stimulants, or herbal preparations (e.g., ephedra, pseudoephedrine, and phenylpropanolamine [PPA]; cathinone in "khat" or *Catha edulis* leaves) also have sympathomimetic activity.

II. PATHOPHYSIOLOGY

A. Sympathomimetics promote the release of and/or block the reuptake of central nervous system (CNS) and sympathetic neurotransmitters, primarily dopamine and norepinephrine, resulting in central and peripheral adrenergic hyperactivity.

B. They also inhibit serotonin reuptake, which may account for their hallucinogenic effects.

C. Sympathomimetics are well absorbed by a variety of routes. Smoking and intravenous (IV) injection of amphetamines produce almost instantaneous effects. Effects occur a few minutes after insufflation and about 30 minutes following ingestion.

  1. Crystallized methamphetamine ("ice") can be smoked.

  2. Abuse of methylphenidate (Ritalin) has occurred through the nasal insufflation of crushed tablets.

D. The plasma half-life of amphetamines varies from 7 to 34 hours (depending on urine flow and urine pH), whereas the half-lives of PPA, ephedrine, and pseudoephedrine are significantly shorter, ranging from 2 to 4 hours.

III. DIAGNOSIS

A. Acute Toxicity

  1. Vital signs may demonstrate tachycardia, hypertension, tachypnea, and hyperthermia.

179

TABLE 33-1	Sympathomimetic Agents

Generic name	Common name
Nonprescription over-the-counter agents	
Phenylpropanolamine	Dexatrim, Comtrex, Allerest
Pseudoephedrine	Sudafed, Novafed
Ephedrine	Primatene, Bronkaid
Propylhexedrine	Benzedrex Inhaler
Desoxyephedrine	Vicks Inhaler
Imidazolines	
Naphazoline	Clear Eyes, Naphcon, Privine
Oxymetazoline	Afrin, Dristan
Tetrahydrozoline	Murine, Visine
Xylometazoline	Otrivin
Prescription (DEA schedule II or III) agents	
Amphetamines	
Methylphenidate	Ritalin
Amphetamine	Adderall
Dextroamphetamine	Dexedrine, Adderall
Phentermine	Fastin, Ionamin

Source: Irwin RS, Rippe JM. *Manual of Intensive Care Medicine,* 3rd ed. Philadelphia: Lippincott Williams & Wilkins, 2000:679.
DEA, Drug Enforcement Administration

2. Additional cardiovascular effects include tachydysrythmias, myocardial infarction, and vasospasm with organ ischemia (e.g., ischemic colitis, renal infarction). Inadvertent intraarterial injection can lead to limb ischemia.

3. CNS effects included agitation, psychosis, seizures, intracerebral hemorrhage, and hyperreflexia.

4. Other effects include diaphoresis, mydriasis, tremor, nausea, rhabdomyolysis, and acute lung injury.

5. Additional toxicity may occur when sympathomimetics are mixed with other agents (e.g., opiates may be injected with amphetamines, known as "speed balling").

B. Chronic Toxicity

1. Valvular heart disease (primarily aortic and mitral regurgitation) has been associated with prolonged (longer than 4 months) and combined usage of the appetite suppressants fenfluramine, dexfenfluramine, and phentermine.

2. Chronic use of amphetamines and 3,4-methylenedioxymethamphetamine (MDMA) has been associated with irreversible damage to CNS dopaminergic and serotonergic neurons.

C. Differential Diagnosis. Anticholinergic intoxication (best distinguished by the absence of diaphoresis), serotonin and withdrawal syndromes,

neuroleptic malignant syndrome, and other nontoxicologic causes of hyper-metabolic states (thyroid dysfunction, pheochromocytoma, heat stroke, infection) should be considered.

D. Evaluation

1. Evaluation should include cardiac monitoring, ECG, complete blood count (CBC), electrolytes, blood urea nitrogen (BUN), creatinine, glucose, and creatine phosphokinase (CPK).
2. Cardiac markers and chest x-ray should be done in patients with an abnormal ECG, cardiac rhythm, or cardiorespiratory complaints or findings.
3. Qualitative urine amphetamine immunoassays can detect most sympathomimetics, although false-positives and false-negatives are frequent.

IV. MANAGEMENT

A. Advanced life support measures should be instituted as necessary.
B. Patients with altered mental status derangement should be initially evaluated by a finger-stick blood glucose to evaluate for hypoglycemia.
C. The mainstay treatment for neuromuscular and cardiovascular stimulation is benzodiazepines. Large doses may be required. If adequate control cannot be quickly achieved, agents such as barbiturates and propofol should be considered (with securing of the airway). Hyperthermia should also be treated with cooling measures.
D. Hypertension and/or significant peripheral vasospasm may be treated with vasodilators such as nitroprusside or phentolamine.
E. Tachydysrhythmias may be treated with propranolol or esmolol.
F. The treatment of myocardial infarction includes benzodiazepines, blood pressure control, and antiplatelet agents. Percutaneous cardiac catheterization and angioplasty appear to be preferable to thrombolysis. Use of β-blockers in this situation is controversial because it may unmask unopposed α-receptor stimulation, resulting in worsening coronary vasospasm.
G. Rhabdomyolysis should be treated with IV fluids and bicarbonate.
H. Activated charcoal should be considered for recent ingestions.
I. Measures to enhance drug elimination are either ineffective (hemodialysis and hemoperfusion) or potentially dangerous (urinary acidification).

V. COMPLICATIONS

A. Complications of acute poisoning include organ ischemia and infarction, cerebral hemorrhage, renal failure from rhabdomyolysis, multiple-organ dysfunction from hyperthermia, and limb ischemia from local injection.
B. Long-term abuse may result in cardiomyopathy, valvulopathy, cerebral vasculitis, or CNS neuronal injury.

Selected Readings

Cho AK. Ice: a new dosage form of an old drug. *Science* 1990;249:631–634.
A review of the history, pharmacology, abuse patterns, and clinical effects of methamphetamine.

Derlet RW, Rice P, Horowitz BZ, et al. Amphetamine toxicity: experience with 127 cases. *J Emerg Med* 1989;7:157–161.
This retrospective review of 127 cases of amphetamine toxicity discusses toxic clinical symptoms, management, and outcomes.

Ginsberg MD, Hertzman M, Schmidt-Nowara WW. Amphetamine intoxication with coagulopathy, hyperthermia, and reversible renal failure. A syndrome resembling heatstroke. *Ann Intern Med* 1970;73:81–85.
A case report and discussion of the similarities of amphetamine intoxication and heatstroke.

Jerrard DA. "Designer drugs"—a current perspective. *J Emerg Med* 1990;8:733–741.
A comprehensive review of "designer drugs," including amphetamines.

Kase CS, Foster TE, Reed JE, et al. Intracerebral hemorrhage and phenylpropanolamine use. *Neurology* 1987;37:399–404.
Two case reports and discussions of intracerebral hemorrhage associated with phenylpropanolamine use.

Klein-Schwartz W, Gorman R, Oderda GM, et al. Central nervous system depression from ingestion of nonprescription eye drops. *Am J Emerg Med* 1984;2:217–218.
Case reports and review of clinical effects and outcomes of ingestion of imidazoline eye drops.

Liebelt EL, Shannon MW. Small doses, big problems: a selected review of highly toxic common medications. *Pediatr Emerg Care* 1993;9:292–297.
This review includes discussion of clinical toxicity of imidazolines in children.

Pentel P. Toxicity of over-the-counter stimulants. *JAMA* 1984;252:1898–1903.
A review of over-the-counter stimulants, including phenylpropanolamine, ephedrine, and pseudoephedrine.

Scandling J, Spital A. Amphetamine-associated myoglobinuric renal failure. *South Med J* 1982;75:237–240.
A case report and discussion of myoglobinuric renal failure after amphetamine ingestion.

Swenson RD, Golper TA, Bennet WM. Acute renal failure and rhabdomyolysis after ingestion of phenylpropanolamine-containing diet pills. *JAMA* 1982;248:1216.
Case reports and discussion of the association of phenylpropanolamine ingestion, acute renal failure, and rhabdomyolysis.

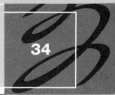

I. BACKGROUND

A. Systemic asphyxiants are chemicals that impair transport of oxygen and/or prevent cellular utilization of oxygen.

B. They include carbon monoxide (CO), cyanide (CN) and cyanogens, hydrogen sulfide (H_2S), and methemoglobin (MetHgb) and sulfhemoglobin (SHgb) inducers.

   1. CO is a colorless, odorless gas produced by the incomplete combustion of fossil fuels and other carbon-containing compounds. It is also produced by the metabolism of methylene chloride (found in paint strippers) and the catabolism of hemoglobin.

   2. CN salts are used in electroplating, metal cleaning and extraction, and laboratory and photographic processes. Cyanide gas (HCN) is released when CN salts are mixed with acids. Cyanogens are compounds that liberate cyanide under certain conditions, such as thermal decomposition (e.g., burning wool, silk, synthetic rubber), hepatic metabolism (e.g., acetonitrile in some artificial nail removers, sodium nitroprusside), or digestion (e.g., laetrile, bitter cassava, peach pits).

   3. H_2S is a colorless, irritating gas with a sulfur or rotten egg odor. It occurs in natural gas, volcanic gas, hot springs, sewer gas, and swampy soils. It is a product of many industrial and manufacturing processes. It may also be formed when acid is added to decaying organic matter as with drain cleaning.

   4. MetHgb inducers include a wide variety of oxidizing agents. Aniline, amino-, nitro-, and nitroso- compounds, antimalarials, dapsone, local anesthetics, nitrates, nitrites, phenazopyridine, and sulfonamides are common offenders.

     a. The MetHgb fraction is normally less than 2%.

     b. Higher fractions are known as methemoglobinemia.

   5. SHgb inducers include many of the medications that cause MetHgb.

II. PATHOPHYSIOLOGY

A. CO has an affinity approximately 250 times greater than that of oxygen for hemoglobin. Binding to hemoglobin produces carboxyhemoglobin (COHgb), which cannot bind oxygen and decreases the oxygen-carrying capacity of the blood. The oxygen–hemoglobin dissociation curve is shifted to the left when COHgb is present, preventing the release of oxygen to tissues. Toxicity may also result from decreased cardiac output and tissue perfusion, binding to intracellular cytochromes, and interference with oxygen utilization.

1. The release of reactive oxygen species from neutrophils adhering to microvascular endothelium may result in reperfusion injury.

2. COHgb is normally present in small amounts (up to 2%).

B. CN binds to the ferric (Fe^{3+}) ion of mitochondrial cytochrome oxidase a_3 thereby inhibiting the formation of adenosine 5'-triphosphate (ATP) in the electron transport chain of the Krebs cycle.

C. The mechanism of H_2S toxicity is the same as that for cyanide.

D. MetHgb inducers oxidize the ferrous (Fe^{2+}) iron in hemoglobin to the non-functional ferric (Fe^{3+} or MetHgb) state, which prevents the binding of oxygen to hemoglobin. The oxygen dissociation curve of MetHgb is also shifted to the left, which decreases oxygen release to tissues. Methemoglobin inducers also variably oxidize hemoglobin protein, with precipitates in red cells (visible as Heinz bodies on peripheral blood smear) and results in splenic degradation (visible as "bite cells" or pie-shaped red cells with a slice missing on peripheral blood smear), and consequent hemolytic anemia.

1. Reduction of Fe^{3+} to Fe^{2+} normally occurs primarily by nicotinamide adenine dinucleotide (NADH)-dependent MetHgb reductase.

2. About 5% occurs via nicotinamide adenine dinucleotide phosphate (NADPH)-dependent MetHgb reductase.

3. Minimal reduction occurs nonenzymatically via ascorbic acid and reduced glutathione, which act as electron donors.

4. Patients with a genetic deficiency of MetHgb reductase and infants (who have decreased enzyme activity) are at increased risk of developing MetHgb.

E. SHgb is functionally similar to MetHgb, but inducing agents bind to hemoglobin at a site other than iron, the oxygen dissociation curve is shifted rightward, and effects are less pronounced than in methemoglobinemia.

F. Regardless of the agent or mechanism involved, the end result is organ, tissue, and cellular hypoxia (systemic asphyxia) and anaerobic metabolism with lactic acidosis.

III. DIAGNOSIS

A. Clinical Toxicity

1. Systemic asphyxia initially stimulates and then depresses vital signs and mental status. Transient tachycardia, hypertension, tachypnea, anxiety, and agitation are followed by cardiovascular, central nervous system (CNS), and respiratory depression.

   a. Symptoms common to all asphyxiants include dizziness, dyspnea, and confusion.

   b. Myocardial ischemia and infarction can occur.

   c. Coma, seizures, syncope, arrhythmias, shock, and metabolic (lactic) acidosis are seen with severe poisoning.

   d. Rapid demise ("knock down" effect) can occur with exposure to high concentrations of asphyxiant gases and with cyanide salt ingestion.

   e. Insidious onset and progression are more typical with ingestions of cyanogens and MetHgb and SHgb inducers.

f. With gases, the severity of poisoning is related to the duration as well as the intensity of exposure (time-concentration or area-under-the curve effect).

g. Patients with anemia are more susceptible to the effects of systemic asphyxiants.

2. CO poisoning usually results from motor vehicle exhaust, home heating systems that burn inefficiently or are poorly ventilated, or smoke inhalation. It can also result from inhalation or ingestion of methylene chloride.

a. Headache, nausea, and vomiting are common.

b. Mild poisoning is usually associated with COHgb fractions of 10% to 30% whereas severe poisoning is usually associated with fractions above 50%.

c. Permanent neurologic damage, ranging from personality changes to encephalopathy, blindness, deafness, seizures, and parkinsonism, can result from severe poisoning.

3. CN poisoning usually occurs in workers with access to cyanide salts who ingest them in a suicide attempt and in victims of fires.

a. Life-threatening toxicity can occur within seconds of HCN inhalation and within 30 minutes of cyanide salt ingestion (200 to 300 mg may be fatal in adults).

b. A bitter almond or musty odor may be present on the breath.

c. Refractory hypotension, pulmonary edema, and profound acidemia are characteristic of severe poisoning.

4. H_2S poisoning primarily results from workplace exposures (natural gas/oil, manure, sewage).

a. Irritant effects may result in tearing, rhinitis, throat pain, cough, and pulmonary edema.

b. The rotten egg odor of H_2S or its ability to cause black discoloration of silver coins and jewelry are diagnostic clues.

5. MetHgb fractions greater than 15% cause cyanosis with a brownish hue.

a. Cyanosis occurs at lower fractions of MetHgb than with deoxyhemoglobin, and patients are less symptomatic than expected for the degree of cyanosis.

b. In contrast to hypoxemic cyanosis, that resulting from MetHgb does not improve with oxygen.

c. Fractions greater than 25% are generally required to produce symptoms.

d. Fractions greater than 50% are associated with severe toxicity.

6. SHgb fractions of only 5% produced cyanosis unresponsive to oxygen, but symptoms are generally mild and rarely life-threatening.

B. Evaluation

1. Evaluation should include cardiac monitoring, oxygen saturation, complete blood count (CBC), electrolytes, blood urea nitrogen (BUN), creatinine, and glucose. Patients with cardiorespiratory signs and symptoms should have an electrocardiogram (ECG) and chest x-ray. Those with a low oxygen saturation or serum bicarbonate should have arterial blood gas measurements taken. A serum lactate level may also be useful.

2. The oxygen saturation (oxyhemoglobin fraction) in CO poisoning and methemoglobinemia and sulfhemoglobinemia is reduced by the fraction

of COHgb/MetHgb/SHgb (and deoxyhemoglobin) present. However, because the pO_2 is normal and most blood gas instruments do not directly measure the oxygen saturation (which requires cooximetry) but report the oxygen saturation calculated from the pO_2, the reported oxygen saturation will be falsely normal. Similarly, although the oxygen saturation measured by pulse oximetry will be low (less than normal and less than that calculated from the pO_2), it will be falsely elevated with respect to the true value (measured by cooximetry). Hence, an "oxygen saturation gap" (a difference between the calculated oxygen saturation and that measured by pulse oximetry) suggests these diagnoses, but the only way to accurately measure the various hemoglobin fractions is by cooximetry, which must be specifically requested. Serial measurements are indicated to evaluate the efficacy of treatment.

3. COHgb fractions must be interpreted with respect to the duration of exposure, time since exposure, and oxygen therapy. Prolonged exposure can result in severe toxicity with fractions of 30% to 50%, and brief exposures with higher fractions may result in minimal symptoms. After exposure is terminated, fractions decline with a half-life of about 4 hours when breathing room air and about 1 hour on 100% oxygen. Hence, the measured COHgb fraction may underestimate the exposure. Clinical evaluation should prevail when making severity assessments.

4. Although whole blood cyanide concentrations can retrospectively confirm cyanide poisoning, they are not readily available to assist with clinical management. Since CN decreases oxygen utilization, the difference between simultaneously obtained arterial and central venous oxygen saturation may be decreased (less than 20%), or the venous PO_2 and oxygen saturation may be increased greater than 40 mm Hg and 70%, respectively).

5. Hydrogen sulfide poisoning can be confirmed only by air sampling.

6. With significant methemoglobinemia, a fresh drop of blood placed on filter paper will appear chocolate-brown in comparison to a control sample. Patients with methemoglobinemia should have serial hematocrit testing to check for hemolysis. A peripheral blood smear, serum haptoglobin, and urinalysis may also be helpful.

7. Most cooximeters are unable to directly quantitate the SHgb fraction, making confirmation unlikely. The fraction can be inferred by subtracting the fractions of measurable hemoglobin species from 100%.

IV. TREATMENT

A. Advanced life support measures should be instituted as necessary.

B. All patients should receive maximal oxygen therapy because oxygen competes with asphyxiant gases for binding sites and provides additional amounts of dissolved oxygen.

C. Seizures may be treated with benzodiazepines and barbiturates.

D. Significant acidemia (serum pH less than 7.2) should be treated with intravenous (IV) sodium bicarbonate.

E. Activated charcoal should be given for recent ingestions (see Chapter 1). Multiples doses (see Chapter 1) can enhance the elimination of dapsone-induced MetHgb, regardless of the time of ingestion.

F. Hyperbaric oxygen (HBO) therapy will shorten the COHgb half-life to about 20 minutes and should be considered for patients with severe CO poisoning or if symptoms persist despite normobaric oxygen therapy. Whether or not HBO prevents permanent neurologic damage remains controversial.

G. CN poisoning is treated with amyl nitrite, sodium nitrite, and sodium thiosulfate. Nitrites promote the formation of MetHgb, which is thought to bind cyanide and promote its release from mitochondrial cytochrome oxidase. Thiosulfate provides substrate for normal detoxification by the enzyme rhodanese (sulfur transferase), which catalyzes the complexing of cyanide with sulfur to form less toxic thiocyanate.

   1. Amyl nitrite pearls can be broken and held under the nose of a spontaneously breathing patient if IV access is delayed.

   2. Otherwise, sodium nitrite is given IV: 300 mg (one 10 mL ampule of 3% solution) is diluted in 100 mL of 0.9% saline and infused over 20 min (10 mg/kg or 0.33 mL/kg up to 300 mg for children).

   3. This is followed by IV sodium thiosulfate: 12.5 g (one 50 mL ampule of 25% solution) for adults, and 1.65 mL/kg up to 50 mL for children.

H. H_2S poisoning unresponsive to oxygen should also be treated with IV sodium nitrite. Resultant MetHgb may bind H_2S and reverse inhibition of cytochrome oxidase. Thiosulfate has no utility, however.

I. HBO should be considered in patients with CN and H_2S poisoning who fail to respond to oxygen and antidotal therapy.

J. Symptomatic patients with methemoglobinemia and those with a MetHgb fraction of 30% or greater should be treated with methylene blue.

   1. Methylene blue can significantly enhance the activity of NADPH-dependent MetHgb reductase.

   2. It is given IV: 1 to 2 mg/kg (0.1 to 0.2 mL/kg of a 1% solution) over 5 min.

   3. The dose may be repeated in 1 hour if improvement is not seen.

   4. The pulse oximeter reading will fall during this treatment because methylene blue absorbs light at the same wavelength that deoxyhemoglobin does.

   5. Methylene blue may not be effective in patients with G-6-PD deficiency because their stores of NADPH (required to activate methylene blue) in red blood cells are decreased.

   6. Exchange transfusion can be performed for severe methemoglobinemia (unresponsive to methylene blue, MetHgb fraction greater than 70%).

   7. The treatment of sulfhemoglobinemia is supportive. Methylene blue is ineffective.

V. COMPLICATIONS

A. Multiple-organ failure may result from severe or prolonged asphyxia.

B. As with CO, victims of severe H_2S poisoning may suffer permanent neurologic damage.

Selected Readings

Beasley DMG, Glass WY. Cyanide poisoning: pathophysiology and treatment recommendations. *Occup Med* 1998;48:427–431.
   Review of the mechanism, clinical features, and treatment of cyanide poisoning.

Beauchamp RO Jr, Bus JS, Popp JA, et al. A critical review of the literature on H₂S toxicity. *Crit Rev Toxicol* 1984;13:25–97.
Discusses the clinical features, pathophysiology, and treatment of hydrogen sulfide poisoning.

Hall AH, Kulig KW, Rumack BH. Drug- and chemical-induced methaemoglobinaemia. Clinical features and management. *Med Toxicol* 1986;1;253–260.
Review of causes, clinical features, pathophysiology, and therapy of methemoglobinemia.

Thom SR, Keim LW. Carbon monoxide poisoning: a review epidemiology, pathophysiology, clinical findings, and treatment options including hyperbaric oxygen therapy. *J Toxicol Clin Toxicol* 1989;27:141–156.
Discusses the causes, clinical features, pathophysiology, and treatment of carbon monoxide poisoning.

Park CM, Nagel RL. Sulfhemoglobinemia: clinical and molecular aspects. *N Engl J Med* 1984;310:1579–1584.
One of the few papers addressing this rare condition.

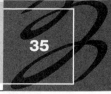

I. BACKGROUND

A. Withdrawal syndromes consist of a constellation of clinical findings in patients who either abruptly discontinue or significantly decrease the dose or frequency of a drug. By definition reinstatement of the drug alleviates the withdrawal syndrome.

B. Withdrawal may develop with many drug classes including ethanol, benzodiazepines (BZDs), barbiturates, other sedative-hypnotics, opioids, γ-hydroxybutyric acid (GHB), antidepressants, and many other agents, including antihypertensive agents, caffeine, and nicotine.

C. Tolerance is a decreased physiologic response to a given dose of drug after chronic administration. Patients who display tolerance are at risk for withdrawal if the drug is discontinued. Other factors increasing the risk, severity, and duration of withdrawal include use of drugs with short duration of effect, high frequency of administration, and long duration of use.

D. Cross-tolerance occurs when the chronic ingestion of one substance decreases the response to another substance. Ethanol, barbiturates, BZDs, and nonbarbiturate–nonbenzodiazepine sedative-hypnotics display cross-tolerance.

II. PATHOPHYSIOLOGY

A. Ethanol

1. During periods of chronic ethanol consumption central nervous system (CNS) sympathetic pathways may counterregulate the sedative effects of ethanol.

2. Cessation of drinking may result in unopposed sympathetic compensatory mechanisms, leading to sympathomimetic excess.

3. Abrupt withdrawal of GABA-potentiating effects of ethanol leads to disinhibition of neural pathways in the CNS.

4. Upregulation of N-methyl D-aspartate (NMDA) receptors, which occurs with chronic intoxication, may contribute to CNS excitation.

B. Sedative-hypnotics

1. BZD tolerance appears to result from the upregulation of BZD receptors. The abundance of unoccupied receptors with drug cessation leads to decreased GABAergic neurotransmission and net CNS excitation.

2. Similar mechanisms likely exist for other sedative-hypnotic drugs, including GHB.

3. Intrathecal baclofen infusion probably results in upregulation of spinal cord GABA-B receptors.

189

C. Opioids
  1. Stimulation of opioid receptors reduces the firing rate of locus ceruleus noradrenergic neurons, resulting in the inhibition of catecholamine release.
  2. Chronic use may produce adrenergic receptor upregulation, leading to increased sympathetic tone with abstinence.

D. Antidepressants. The mechanism of withdrawal is unknown but may involve a rapid decline in serotonergic (and adrenergic) neurotransmission.

III. DIAGNOSIS

A. Clinical Syndromes
  1. Ethanol
    a. Withdrawal produces a hyperadrenergic state characterized by intense sympathetic nervous system activation. Manifestations include tachycardia, hypertension, tremors, seizures, and delirium.
    b. Tremors occur early and are signs of mild to moderate withdrawal. They begin 6 to 8 hours after a reduction in ethanol intake and may occur despite detectable serum ethanol concentrations of 100 mg/dL. Other symptoms in this phase include nausea, vomiting, anorexia, anxiety, and insomnia, which peak between 24 and 36 hours. Recovery occurs within a few days. About 20% to 25% of these patients progress to more serious symptoms.
    c. Most ethanol withdrawal seizures occur within 7 to 48 hours of cessation or relative abstinence. They may occur after the onset of mild withdrawal symptoms or herald the onset of withdrawal. They are short, generalized, tonic–clonic seizures. Forty percent are isolated. If they recur it is generally within a few hours of the first occurrence. Status epilepticus is rare. The occurrence of seizures does suggest a higher incidence of severe withdrawal, including delirium tremens.
    d. The hallmark of delirium tremens is a significant alteration of sensorium associated with dramatic autonomic and CNS hyperactivity. This is rarely seen before 48 to 72 hours after cessation of ethanol and may be delayed up to 5 to 14 days. Patients are disoriented and display global confusion, hallucinations, delusions, mumbling speech, and psychomotor agitation. Tachycardia, hypertension, hyperpyrexia, diaphoresis, and mydriasis are present.
    e. Alcoholic hallucinosis occurs in a small subset of individuals and consists of hallucinations, typically disabling auditory hallucinations, in the absence of tremor or autonomic findings. It occurs within 8 to 48 hours of cessation and generally lasts 1 to 6 days. Rare cases persist for months.
  2. Benzodiazepines
    a. Signs of BZD withdrawal are similar to those from ethanol.
    b. Unlike ethanol, the time of symptom onset depends on the particular medication. Short-acting drugs such as alprazolam cause symptom onset within hours of discontinuation, whereas diazepam withdrawal may not develop for days.

3. Barbiturate and nonbenzodiazepine–nonbarbiturate sedative-hypnotics
   a. Withdrawal is generally similar to that from ethanol.
   b. Chronic delivery of baclofen through an intrathecal pump for spastic neuromuscular disorders may be interrupted when the infusion becomes disconnected or the medication runs out. Marked muscle rigidity is seen with this method. Withdrawal from orally dosed baclofen is uncommon.
4. GHB
   a. Withdrawal is generally similar to that from ethanol.
   b. Users of GHB typically dose the drug every 1 to 2 hours, including awakening at night for administration. Therefore, symptom onset is much more rapid than with other sedatives.
5. Opioids
   a. Early signs of opioid withdrawal include mydriasis, lacrimation, rhinorrhea, diaphoresis, yawning, piloerection, anxiety, and restlessness. This may progress to mild elevation of pulse and blood pressure as well as the development of myalgias, vomiting, diarrhea, anorexia, abdominal pain, and dehydration. Intense drug craving is unique to opioid withdrawal.
   b. Heroin withdrawal begins within 4 to 8 hours of the last dose, whereas withdrawal from methadone occurs after 36 to 72 hours.
   c. Unlike ethanol or sedative withdrawal, opioid withdrawal is not life-threatening because patients do not have altered mental status, hyperthermia, and seizures. The exception is neonatal withdrawal, which may involve seizures and is life-threatening.
6. Antidepressants
   a. Withdrawal from any antidepressant, but particularly short-acting selective serotonin reuptake inhibitors (paroxetine), may cause symptoms of nausea, headaches, restlessness, and fatigue.
   b. Signs and symptoms are not life-threatening.

B. Evaluation
   1. Perform a complete physical examination.
   2. Check vital signs for hyperpyrexia, tachycardia, and hypertension.
   3. Examine for signs of trauma, infection, and focal neurologic deficits.
   4. Evaluate for metabolic derangements, particularly with alcoholics.
      a. Obtain a complete blood count (CBC), electrolytes (including Ca^{2+}, Mg^{2+}, Phos), blood urea nitrogen (BUN), creatinine, creatine phosphokinase (CPK), glucose, and liver function tests (LFTs).
      b. Consider cranial computed tomography (CT) and lumbar puncture to rule out CNS trauma or infection.

C. Differential Diagnosis
   1. The differential diagnosis for withdrawal includes all other causes of a hyperadrenergic state, including hypoglycemia, sympathomimetic drugs such as amphetamines, serotonin syndrome, neuroleptic malignant syndrome, and underlying metabolic, infectious, or traumatic disorders.
   2. Consider the possibility of intracranial hemorrhage, meningitis, encephalitis, hypoxia, sepsis, thiamine deficiency, thyroid storm, pheochromocytoma, and hepatic encephalopathy.

IV. TREATMENT

A. General Principles

1. Anticipation and recognition of early signs of ethanol and sedative-hypnotic withdrawal allow timely treatment and prevent the development of serious manifestations such as seizures, hyperthermia, and delirium.
2. In general, treatment relies on replacement therapy with cross-tolerant drugs that alleviate symptoms and can be tapered.
3. Tapering should generally occur over 2 to 4 weeks (e.g., by decreasing the dose 10% to 20% every 3 days).
4. Management includes treatment of coexisting medical problems.

B. Ethanol

1. Use withdrawal assessment tools to grade severity and guide therapy.
2. The Clinical Institute Withdrawal Assessment (CIWA) scale provides a numbered grading system based on the patient's mental status (e.g., reported anxiety, hallucinations, disorientation). Scores are used to determine the need for sedation with BZDs.
3. Achievement of adequate sedation (sleeping, yet arousable) is the cornerstone of therapy. BZDs have proved the most effective.
   a. Long-acting BZDs with active metabolites (diazepam or chlordiazepoxide) offer a prolonged therapeutic effect without the need for frequent dosing.
   b. IV therapy can be followed with oral dosing.
   c. Initial doses of 5 to 20 mg IV diazepam every 5 minutes are given until sleep is induced.
   d. Some patients require very high doses (up to 1,000 mg diazepam in 24 h).
4. Barbiturates act synergistically with BZD at GABA receptors.
   1. Pentobarbital in increments of 100 mg can be given orally or IV for severe withdrawal that is unresponsive to BZDs.
   2. Barbiturates have a poor safety profile in nonintubated patients because of the risk of respiratory depression.
5. In intubated patients, IV propofol (direct GABA effect) can also be used for severe withdrawal unresponsive to BZD.
6. Phenothiazines (prochlorperazine, chlorpromazine) and butyrophenones (haldol) lower the seizure threshold, induce hypotension, impair thermoregulation, and should be avoided.
7. Other therapies include initial administration of thiamine 100 mg, folate 1 mg, and a multivitamin. Alert patients may take these orally. Magnesium replacement is also warranted because many alcoholics have low Mg^{2+} stores.

C. Sedative-hypnotics

1. Dose requirements for patients with physical dependence on BZDs and barbiturates are generally far lower than those for alcohol withdrawal.
2. Reinstituting the withdrawn medication at previously used doses is generally sufficient to alleviate symptoms.
3. Cross-tolerant medications may be used (e.g., BZD for barbiturate withdrawal).

4. As with ethanol withdrawal, neuroleptic medications have no role in therapy.

5. GHB withdrawal may also be treated with BZDs, although there is evidence that barbiturates are more effective. Initial doses of a short-acting barbiturate such as pentobarbital can be given IV (50 to 150 mg every 15 min) until mild sedation is achieved. This can be followed by oral dosing with a long-acting barbiturate such as phenobarbital (one-third the effective dose of IV pentobarbital, or usually 30 to 60 mg) every 8 hours.

6. Baclofen withdrawal should be treated by reinstituting the previous dose of baclofen.

D. Opioids

1. Withdrawal may be treated either with long-acting opioids (e.g., sustained-release oxycodone or methadone) or medications that blunt the sympathetic response to withdrawal (e.g., clonidine).

   a. An initial dose of 20 mg methadone by mouth (PO) daily will generally relieve most symptoms but may not curb drug cravings.

   b. Clonidine 0.2 to 0.3 mg PO three times a day may alleviate some of the autonomic symptoms but not drug craving.

   c. Dosing of opioids or clonidine can be tapered over several days.

2. In the United States, treatment of opioid addiction with methadone requires that the facility be licensed for such treatment by the Food and Drug Administration (FDA), Drug Enforcement Administration (DEA), and designated state authorities. This does not preclude nonlicensed facilities from treating opioid withdrawal in patients who are admitted for other reasons.

E. Antidepressants

1. Reinstituting the previous dosage of the withdrawn agent is sufficient to alleviate symptoms.

2. The medication can then be tapered over 2 to 3 weeks.

V. COMPLICATIONS include those related to withdrawal (e.g., dehydration, electrolyte disturbances, hyperthermia, rhabdomyolysis, seizures, aspiration), its treatment (e.g., CNS and respiratory depression, aspiration), and underlying illness (e.g., infection, nutritional deficiencies, trauma).

Selected Readings

Ritson B, Chick J. Comparison of two benzodiazepines in the treatment of alcohol withdrawal: effects on symptoms and cognitive recovery. *Drug Alcohol Depend* 1986;18:329–334.
   This paper discusses the preferential use of long-acting benzodiazepines with active metabolites (diazepam), rather than short-acting BZDs without active metabolites (lorazepam), in the treatment of ethanol withdrawal.

Sivilotti ML, Burns MJ, Aaron CK, et al. Pentobarbital for severe gamma-butyrolactone withdrawal. *Ann Emerg Med* 2001;38:660–665.
   This case series illustrates the features of GHB withdrawal and demonstrates the effectiveness of barbiturates compared with BZDs for treating symptoms.

Note: Page numbers followed by f indicate illustrations; those followed by t indicate tables.

A

Acebutolol, 71t. *See also* β-blockers
Acetaminophen poisoning, 14–17
Acetone, serum osmolality and, 5t
Acetylcholinesterase inhibitors
    for neuromuscular blocker poisoning, 153
    poisoning by, 80–83
N-Acetylcysteine
    for acetaminophen poisoning, 15–17
    for mercury poisoning, 119
Acid-base disturbances
    in salicylate poisoning, 156, 156t
    in withdrawal syndromes, 191
Acid injuries, 88–91, 121–125
Acrodynia, 118
Activated charcoal, 9. *See also specific poisons*
    antiemetics with, 147
    multiple-dose, 11
Acute dystonic reactions, 66, 68
Acyclovir poisoning, 59, 61–62
Advanced life support. *See specific poisons*
Agkistrodon envenomations, 101–103
Akathisia, from antipsychotics, 66, 68
Alcoholic hallucinosis, 190
Alcoholic ketoacidosis, 20, 21
Alcohol poisoning, 19–22
    serum osmolality and, 5t
Alcohol withdrawal, 189–193
Aleplon poisoning, 174–178
Alkali ingestions, 88–91
Alkaline diuresis therapy, for salicylate poisoning, 158, 158t
Alkalinization, urinary, 11
    for salicylate poisoning, 158, 158t
Alkalosis, in salicylate poisoning, 156, 156t
A₁ receptor antagonists
    dosing guidelines for, 53t
    poisoning by, 50–52, 55
    preparations of, 53t

Alpidem poisoning, 174–178
Aluminum poisoning, from pesticides, 165–168
Amantadine
    for neuroleptic-induced parkinsonism, 68
    poisoning by, 59, 61–62
Amiloride
    dosing guidelines for, 50t
    poisoning by, 47, 55
Aminoglycoside poisoning, 59, 61–62
Amiodarone poisoning, 24–29
Amisulpride, 64t. *See also* Antipsychotics
Amitriptyline poisoning, 41–46
Amlodipine poisoning, 76
Ammonium fluoride poisoning, 121
Amoxapine poisoning, 41–46
Amphetamine poisoning, 179–182
Amphotericin B poisoning, 60, 61–62
Amrinone, for calcium channel blocker poisoning, 77
Amyl nitrite, for cyanide poisoning, 187
Anesthetics
    abuse of, 170–173
    local, 142–144, 183–189
    malignant hypertension and, 153
    sedative-hypnotic
        poisoning by, 174–178
        reversal of, 178
Angiotensin-converting enzyme (ACE) inhibitors
    dosing guidelines for, 51t
    poisoning by, 50, 55
    preparations of, 51t
Angiotensin-II receptor antagonists
    dosing guidelines for, 52t
    poisoning by, 50, 55
    preparations of, 52t
Aniline poisoning, 183–187
Anion gap, in diagnosis, 2, 5f